CRADLED *on* BOTH SIDES

Bearing Witness at the Thresholds of Life

LEANN THRAPP

LEGACY press

Published by Legacy Press
LegacyPress.org
Your life tells a story; we can help you write it.

Author's Note on Privacy: This book is a work of creative nonfiction. It reflects true experiences from my life and work, shared with care and integrity.

To protect privacy and honor confidentiality, certain names, identifying details, and scenes have been changed. This includes patients, families, and personal relationships. These changes were made intentionally and ethically, in keeping with my responsibilities as a healthcare provider and my respect for those whose stories intersect with mine.

While some details have been altered, the emotional truth of each experience remains.

Printed in the United States of America

ISBN (print): 978-1-957026-43-5
ISBN (eBook): 978-1-957026-44-2

Manuscript development and writing support by Robin Grunder: *robingrunder.org*
Edited by Abbi Beckett: *abbibeckett.com*
Cover design and interior formatting by Nelly Murariu: *pixbeedesign.com*

Dedication

For my parents, who gave me life, endurance, and the quiet belief that I could do hard things.

CONTENTS

INTRODUCTION

This is not a gentle book.

It is honest. It is raw. Some of my stories may be hard to read because they were hard to live through. For more than forty years, I stood at bedsides from birth to death, cradling life as it arrived and as it let go. Along the way, I carried my own fractures, fears, and failures, often quietly, often alone.

There was a time when my life looked nothing like it was "supposed" to. I was working three jobs, raising my son, and barely scraping by. I didn't feel aligned. I didn't feel settled. And yet, somehow, through the grit of family, the kindness of strangers, and moments of grace I didn't recognize until later, things slowly began to fall into place.

When I first sat down to write, I thought I was writing a kind of guidebook. The things they never told us in nursing school. The things they should have taught us. After decades in high-risk obstetrics, labor and delivery, and hospice, I believed I could gather what mattered most. I have lectured, mentored, and even written for nursing textbooks, but there were still truths that lived between the lines.

Because for all the classes and clinicals, no one prepared me for what it feels like to sit in a room where a life has just ended—or begun. No one taught us what to say when a family looks into your eyes, searching for comfort you don't know how to give. No one told us how heavy silence can feel, or how sacred it can be.

I thought I was writing down lessons. Practical wisdom for nurses, for students, for anyone stepping into the clinic, hospital, or the hospice room. But as the words came, I realized they weren't lessons at all. They were stories. My stories. Stories of patients and families, of mistakes and miracles, of moments that broke me open and others that stitched me back together. Stories that weren't meant to be bullet points in a lecture, but the living pulse of a life spent at the thresholds of birth and death.

And if my career taught me anything, it is this: we can master procedures, memorize diagnoses, publish and teach and carry every credential after our name, and still be unprepared for the moment a child takes her last breath, or a family turns to you in their undoing.

Somewhere along the way, the book shifted. It stopped being just about what I had learned for others, and it became about who I had become. The stories that shaped me. The griefs I carried quietly for years. The healing I never expected to find. What began as a teaching tool became a memoir. What I thought was for students became a legacy—for my colleagues, yes, but also for the families I've met, and for anyone who has ever been asked to sit in the sacred space of loss.

This book may resonate with nurses, but it's not only for them. It's for daughters and sons, mothers and fathers, caregivers and friends. It's for anyone who has ever stood in a doorway—wondering if they've missed some invisible instruction manual—unsure of how to stay present when everything in them wanted to run.

And so, I invite you into my story. In truth, our stories never start only with us—they begin in the hush of voices we never heard, generations before we were even thought of. Still, every life, every story, has its own threshold, its own first room.

For me, that room was 107.

PROLOGUE
ROOM 107

I was sixteen the first time I sat with someone who was dying. It happened in Room 107.

The air felt heavy, like the room itself was holding its breath. A fan hummed steadily, moving the curtain just enough to pulse with the air. The sheet lifted barely over the man's chest—fluttering like it, too, was preparing to leave. His breaths were shallow, slow, each one a fragile thread between staying and going.

"Just sit with Ed. He doesn't have long," my nursing supervisor instructed.

I sat at the end of his bed, not to be close, but so I could see the hallway—life moving on just beyond the door. I was terrified that if I looked directly at him, he might stop breathing. That death might notice me noticing it.

I was a certified nursing assistant in a nursing home, and I had just learned how to take a pulse. No one had ever taught me how to sit with the dying. Nurses taught charts, not silence. Teachers taught CPR, not how to say goodbye. So I sat quietly, hands folded, waiting for someone to tell me what came next.

Ed didn't die while I was there. Not that day. But something in me changed in that room. It was the first time I brushed against death, the first time I felt the unspoken weight of grief. I carried it out with me, folded into a quiet corner of myself, and, as I'd learned to do in so many areas of my life, I simply carried on as though nothing happened.

Looking back, I see how that moment planted a seed. I didn't know it then, but Room 107 would become the place I kept circling back to. The place that taught me presence matters more than performance. The place that would eventually send me back into hospital rooms and hospice rooms, to sit with strangers at the edge of life—the beginning and the end—and learn the lesson I first felt at sixteen: *silence speaks, and presence heals.*

PART I

BECOMING (UN)PREPARED

The caterpillar begins in silence,
carrying more than it knows, preparing
for a change it cannot yet imagine.

CHAPTER 1

BEFORE THE BEDSIDE

When I was young, silence was the language of survival.

We didn't talk about grief. We didn't talk about love either—not out loud. I don't remember my parents saying, *I love you.* They may have, but I don't remember it. Love wasn't spoken in our house—it was lived, imperfectly and quietly. A car appearing before prom night. Mom's busy hands cooking and cleaning. Love was always there, but it was wordless.

We also didn't talk about the darker things.

Dad's binge drinking. His blackouts. Mom's black eyes explained away as "just an elbow." The nights he fumbled shells into a gun while I stood between them, begging him to take it out on me instead. The times we both packed up into the car only to turn back, whispering vows about "for better or for worse."

Our table often had an empty chair, waiting for Dad. Sometimes we sat there until what seemed like midnight. Eventually, we stopped waiting.

That was the inheritance I didn't know I was carrying: love without words, pain without naming, survival without speaking. I didn't know yet how much of that silence had been handed down, long before it reached me. It shaped me. It prepared me—and unprepared me—for what was ahead. It taught me to keep my guard up, to wear a mask, to keep moving as though nothing happened.

But grief doesn't disappear just because no one names it. It hides. It festers. It becomes the shadow we drag behind us.

But grief doesn't disappear just because no one names it. It hides. It festers. It becomes the shadow we drag behind us.

Still, there was another inheritance, too.

I was a happy third-born child, drawn to the outdoors. We lived near a small river, and I loved the path we wore through the grass from our house to the water. We had mud fights until our skin was stained brown, rode bikes until our legs burned, roller-skated, played softball, and tumbled down snowy hills on sleds. Life in the 1960s was simple for my two brothers and sister and me—we didn't have much, but we never went without.

I loved birthdays—not just my own, but celebrating others. Buying gifts, making them, wrapping them with care—it was my way of speaking love out loud. I sewed and crafted constantly, often working on Christmas gifts months in advance, my hands busy long before the season arrived. I kept scrapbooks, tie-dyed crafts, and even a bug collection. I cared for guppies and cheered when they had babies. I had four living great-grandparents and spent many weekends visiting them, growing up in the rare company of four generations.

There were times I needed escape. After we moved to the farm, life grew heavier. Dad seemed angrier, and we all walked on eggshells. My sister Tammy and I fought constantly as sisters tend to do; my only goal was to beat her at everything, and I usually did. When it felt like too much, I hid in my tidy room, arranging my favorite treasures, or escaped to my cousin Robyn's house, where we ran through our chores so we could go to our happy place, the swimming pool. Those were places of quiet relief, where the air wasn't so thick with tension, at least not the kind I could name.

But silence was still the rule of our house. We didn't speak of the things that hurt. We didn't name what frightened us. I remember being terrified when my younger brother got lost at the fair, or later, when Mom had an appendicitis attack. I was only fifteen, driving on a permit, when I had to take her into Iowa City myself. Dad was in the field, unwilling—or unable—to climb down from the tractor, and his response was simply, "Well, take her then," as if her pain wasn't reason enough for him to stop. The only car at home was my oldest brother Jay's, a car we loved but were never allowed to drive. I knew he would be furious. Still, it was the only transportation Mom and I had. I drove through city streets I'd never seen before, hands shaking on the wheel, praying she would survive.

There were small lessons in silence, too. As a toddler, I was bitten regularly by a little girl. Her mother urged me to bite back, but I refused. I endured it until one day, that same mother bit her own daughter to make her stop. The biting ended, but the lesson lingered: I would not fight back, even when wronged. I carried that forward, telling myself, *God knows. I don't need to say a word.*

All of this—mud fights and empty chairs, laughter and fear, silence and survival—wove together into the girl I was becoming. A girl who longed to be seen by her father, scanning the bleachers at every softball game, just in case he showed up. A girl who knew joy and love, but only in whispers and actions, never in words.

I didn't know it then, but those years were shaping me for the bedside. They were teaching me to notice what wasn't spoken. To read the air in a room. To carry on as though nothing happened—even when everything had.

But silence has a way of following you. It trailed me out of childhood and into the choices I made as a young woman. Some silences you inherit. Others you choose.

And one silence I carried would change everything.

CHAPTER 2

THE PREGNANCY I HID

By the time I was seventeen, silence had become second nature. It seemed almost normal to keep secrets tucked away, to live with what was hidden. So when I found myself carrying a child, I did what I had always done: I covered it.

I wore the same oversized blouse, a red one that became my shield. Fabric did the work my voice could not. My body was telling the truth, but I had no language for it. My periods had never been regular, so I told myself it wasn't possible. I didn't let myself imagine a baby growing inside me, even when I knew.

The first moment it truly hit me was ordinary—I was sitting in the bathtub, staring down at my belly, when I felt it deep in my bones: *I am pregnant.* That same day, Mom asked me if I was "in trouble." I whispered yes. She didn't scold me or collapse in despair. Instead, she laid out three choices—abortion, adoption, or keeping the baby. I was already too far along for abortion, and truthfully, I knew I couldn't do that anyway. Still, I was so disconnected from my body, from what was growing inside me, that when I answered, I said, "I'm keeping it." Not because my baby was an *it*, but because I didn't yet have words for the life I was carrying. And with that, the path was set.

There was no real conversation about expectations with the baby's father. No proposal. In 1979, a girl in my shoes didn't weigh her options. She just got married. So I sewed my own wedding dress and the bridesmaid dresses too, stitches of shame and duty instead of lace and joy. At eighteen I walked down the aisle into a marriage I already knew wouldn't last.

There should have been flowers, dreams of the future, celebrating new life. Instead, it felt like a smoothing-over, a way to make my silence more presentable. Somehow, a wedding made it all look "better," even if everyone knew the truth.

I tried to disappear. I worked nights at the hospital in Washington, Iowa, hiding the pregnancy as long as I could. Sleeping during the day and working in the dark made me invisible. I numbed myself with busyness, pretending nothing was happening, even as life was unfolding inside me.

I numbed myself with busyness, pretending nothing was happening, even as life was unfolding inside me.

When the time came, I drove myself to the hospital in a February snowstorm. My baby's father lost his license, so I gripped the wheel and prayed my way across icy roads. I realized as I pulled into the parking lot that I had come full circle—back to the same hospital where, at fifteen, I had once driven my mother in an emergency. Only now, it was my own body in crisis, and I was terrified.

The labor was long, induced, and grueling. The nurses treated me like I was less than, their glances sharp, their care dismissive—as if being young and presumed unwed made me undeserving of tenderness. But my physician was different. He was steady, calm, and kind. At one point, he went to fetch my mom and asked her to come tell me to relax, a simple act that soothed my fear more than any drug could.

I remember the moment my baby's heart rate dropped, the monitor dipping into danger. The doctor's voice was firm: "It's time to have this baby." They rushed me to the delivery room.

The cord was wrapped around his neck and body, and every push felt like a battle. Push. Stop. Push again. I followed every instruction, heart pounding, until finally—he was here.

He was red, floppy, and quiet.

And then came the cry.

Thin. Wobbly. Alive.

That sound was my salvation. In that cry, I knew I was not lost.

For five days, I held him in awe, staring at his tiny body, whispering promises I didn't yet know how to keep. I remember looking at him and thinking, *How will I ever care for you when I can't even care for myself?*

But something fierce rose up in me—something older than silence, stronger than shame. His name was Jared. He became my reason. My anchor. My voice.

Those early months were hard beyond words. I worked constantly—days at the university, nights and weekends at the county hospital, and waitressing in between. Jared's father didn't work, disappearing on weekends with friends, leaving me to stretch myself thin. Thank God for Mom and Dad, for my sister, Tammy, and brother, Gary, who helped me carry what I could not. And thank God for my Grandma Pearl Richardson—my confidant, my protector, my safe place. She never judged me, only loved me. Her forgiveness was the kind that covered me when nothing else could.

The world judged me harshly. Nurses dismissed my questions. Community whispers stung. But I found that I didn't care anymore—not the way I once had. Judgment faded into background noise. I had a child to raise, a life to protect, and that life mattered more than what anyone thought of me.

Looking back, I see a generational thread that connects us. My grandmother was only eighteen when she carried my father, hidden away in a home for unwed mothers. Her pregnancy was never spoken of; her labor and delivery happened alone, behind closed doors. My father was born into silence, carried home without welcome, without words. He never spoke of those beginnings, but I wonder if that absence of acknowledgment was etched into him, shaping the father he would become.

And then there was me, eighteen and hiding a pregnancy of my own. Without realizing it, I was carrying not just my secret, but hers too. Three generations bound together by the same silence, the same unspoken shame.

But when Jared was born, that pattern broke. His first cry filled the room with sound that could not be ignored. What had been hidden for generations was, in that moment, announced.

Silence had been my inheritance. Jared became my turning point.

CHAPTER 3

BLOOD ON THE FLOOR

Silence followed me everywhere. I carried it out of childhood and into my marriage. By nineteen, that marriage was already unraveling, and I was in the process of divorce. I carried silence through the long nights of rocking my son, when love and shame kept me equally awake. And I carried it with me into the hospital, where grief lived under fluorescent lights but was never named.

At home, silence had been survival. In marriage, silence became resignation. At work, silence became an expectation. In medicine, there are things we don't talk about—not the weight of loss, not the ache that lingers, not the faces that follow you home.

Hospitals have their own rhythm—the steady beeping of monitors, the shuffle of shoes across polished tile, the sharp tang of antiseptic clinging to everything. I was still new enough to be learning its beat, falling in step with the constant urgency, when one day the pattern broke.

The intercom crackled overhead: "Two traumas, incoming!"

The room lurched out of rhythm, like a sudden arrhythmia in a once-steady heart. Doors slammed open. Voices rose. A young man, not much older than I was, came flying through the doorway of Room Six. The team surged around him, instruments clattering, orders flying, blood spilling faster than I could take it in. I looked for my trainer, but she wasn't there. I was alone, trying to keep up, terrified of doing something wrong.

And then—silence.

Just like that, it was over.

The urgency drained from the room as staff walked away one by one. The young man lay exposed under the lights—no sheet, no covering, no dignity. His body still. The room stripped of motion.

I wanted to cover him. I wanted to shield his body from the harshness of fluorescent light and cold tile. But I didn't move.

The clinical nurse specialist came in, calm as ever. She began counting instruments, as though nothing had happened. She looked at me and said, "I think you probably need to vacuum first, Leann."

So I did.

I walked carefully through the blood pooled on the floor, pulled the suction hose from the wall, and began. The sound filled the room—like the hollow hum of a dentist's suction, only louder, more violent. I sprayed the floor, vacuumed again, methodical, mechanical, mindless. I put the hose back in the wall and stood up, lightheaded, sweaty, and shaky.

She smiled at me. "Sometimes this happens. You did an amazing job today."

I nodded.

But I didn't feel amazing. I felt like running. I felt like crying. I felt like throwing up. Instead, I peeled off my gown, hair cover, gloves, and bloody shoe covers, washed my hands, and went to lunch with the others.

We talked about weekend plans. I remember thinking, *How does anyone eat after that?* But we did. Because that's what the job required. Because no one told us how not to.

You just carry on—as though nothing happened.

That phrase followed me everywhere.

It echoed the silence I already knew at home: the black eyes explained away, the empty chair at the table, the nights pretending nothing was wrong. It echoed the silence of my hidden pregnancy: wearing the same shirt, sewing a wedding dress for a marriage I knew was crumbling. And now, it echoed in the silence of medicine: blood on the floor, a mother somewhere about to get a call that would break her, and the rest of us going to lunch like nothing had happened.

This was where my two worlds collided. The silence I had inherited at home now met the silence of the hospital. Both demanded that I carry on, even when everything inside me was breaking. Both taught me that grief had no place at the table.

My training had taught me how to calculate dosages, how to prep a room, how to follow protocols. But it hadn't taught me how to stand in the stillness of grief. It hadn't prepared me for the weight of presence—the way silence can either wound or heal, depending on how you hold it.

Silence can either wound or heal, depending on how you hold it.

On long drives home, I cried the tears I couldn't shed under fluorescent lights. My chest tight, my stomach knotted, my whole body aching with something I didn't have words for. I thought it was nerves or stress. But it was grief. My body knew what my mind refused to admit: this mattered. This death mattered. And pretending it didn't was eating me alive.

Looking back, I see now: the hospital wasn't just training me as a nurse. It was teaching me a language I already knew too well—how to keep going when your insides are falling apart. But here, for the first time, I began to sense something different stirring beneath the silence. A whisper of presence. A call to name grief instead of hiding it.

Because in the end, it wasn't the blood on the floor that stayed with me—it was the silence that followed, and the realization that no textbook could prepare me for what to do in that silence.

Skills could teach me how to calculate a drip rate or start an IV, but they couldn't teach me how to stand still in the presence of death. They couldn't teach me how to carry the weight of grief without turning away.

That was something I would only learn by being there. By staying. By realizing that presence itself could be medicine.

CHAPTER 4

THE GUARD

The silence I carried out of that trauma room didn't leave me. It settled into me, pressing against the places too raw to name. Being present in the stillness of this loss of life had left me shaken, so I did what felt safe: I began to guard myself. Guard my words. Guard my feelings. Guard the parts of me that felt too tender to reveal. If I couldn't change the silence around me, I could at least control the silence within me.

By the time I was working as a nursing assistant in the operating room, I had learned how to live this way—behind the practiced calm, the *everything-is-fine* face. It was survival, though I didn't call it that at the time. I only knew that if I stayed guarded, I couldn't be caught off balance.

Part of my role was transporting patients to and from surgery. Most days, I loved it. It let me step out from behind the sterile masks and instruments, if only for a short walk down a corridor. But even then, I stayed guarded. Professional. Polite. Careful not to let anyone see what was happening inside me.

One day I was sent to pick up a patient from C-22 on the second floor. The patient was already waiting on the gurney when I returned with the chart—quiet beneath a crisp white sheet. I wheeled the gurney through the ward, the shuffle of slippers and the hum of machines filling the air. As I began to wheel him toward the elevator, a man walked alongside us. He was calm, watchful. I assumed he was family, keeping company as far as he could before letting go.

At the elevator, I told him visitors couldn't go any further. He nodded, turned, and walked away without protest. The elevator was one of the old ones, with a heavy metal door and an inner scissor gate that clanged loudly when I pulled it open. I rolled the patient inside and pressed the button for the sixth floor. He never once looked at me—not even a glance. Most patients sought something before surgery—reassurance, connection, a shared breath of courage. But he stayed silent, closed off, unreachable. I remember standing beside him, unsure how to bridge the quiet, wishing I knew how.

When the doors screeched open on the sixth floor, I pushed the gurney out—and froze. The same man I had told to stay behind was already there, waiting for us. Calm. Composed. As if he had never left.

At the OR desk, I slid the stamper card through the slot, and waited at the glass window. Still, he hovered close. I whispered nervously to my trainer, "I told him he couldn't come on the elevator. But here he is."

She gave me a knowing smile then pointed at the chart. "Look at the address," she said.

I glanced down. The address was for the state penitentiary.

"That's not a guest," she said. "That's the guard."

I stared at her, suddenly aware of the weight of what had just happened. The man lying silently on the gurney beside me was not just any patient—he was a prisoner, a violent offender, shackled beneath that crisp white sheet. And the "family member" was a corrections officer, silently performing his role, ensuring security without drawing attention.

The sheet had hidden more than chains—it had masked the truth of the moment. The convict never looked at me because he knew I didn't know. And I think now, his silence—his refusal to meet my eyes—wasn't fear or defiance. It was restraint. Maybe even mercy. That kind of stillness people carry when they're used to others assuming they've done something wrong. He didn't look at me because he thought I knew what I was doing. Or maybe because he knew I didn't.

And the truth is—no one taught me how to do this part. No one taught me that behind a white sheet could be more than a nervous patient. No one taught me that sometimes the most important details are the quiet ones: an address, a look not exchanged, a silence that holds a warning.

Sometimes the most important details are the quiet ones.

From that moment on, I checked the address. Every time. And from that moment on, I never questioned when a "guest" stepped into the elevator with us.

Because sometimes, the guest isn't a guest at all—they're the guard.

And sometimes, the guard isn't outside of us. Sometimes the guard is the one we station inside—quietly keeping watch, keeping us safe, but also keeping us from being fully seen.

At home, silence had taught me to survive. In the hospital, it threatened to undo me. So I learned to meet it with armor. I guarded myself carefully—my words, my feelings, the parts of me that felt too raw to reveal—believing it was the only way to keep going.

The guard might be able to keep us steady—but if we're not careful, it can also keep us numb.

CHAPTER 5

THE MEMORY AND THE MISTAKE

I'd once taken a class on death and dying. At twenty-two, it felt out of place in a curriculum built around saving lives. We were supposed to fight illness, restore health, keep death at bay—not study it. I remembered the name of the woman we read about, Elisabeth Kübler-Ross, and how she spoke of dying as a natural part of living. I didn't understand her then. I only knew I wanted no part of it.

And yet here I was, standing at the doorway of the medical intensive care unit.

I paused there for a moment, letting the hum of machines and the faint antiseptic scent settle around me before taking another step. I was in my final quarter of nursing school, and I was about to begin my Medical Intensive Care Unit rotation—surrounded by patients whose lives hung in the balance, their breathing now the job of machines. The moment I crossed the threshold, time folded in on itself and a memory rose up to meet me.

Ten beds lined the ward, five on each side, separated by striped curtains. The place was loud, bright, relentless. Monitors beeped, ventilators hissed, IV pumps clicked like clocks. The air smelled of sickness and bleach.

Years earlier, my great-aunt Mick—my grandmother Dorothy's sister—had been in a head-on collision and landed in this same MICU. She adored my father, fiercely protective of him, and often told me I reminded her of my grandmother. I remember the chaos—the sharp beeping of monitors, the hiss of suction, and my father's voice calling her name. She hadn't moved in days, but somehow, when he spoke, her toe flicked beneath the white sheet. He was the only one she responded to. For a breath, it felt like hope. Mostly, I felt relief—that we could leave, that she was still on this side of the curtain.

I can still see that image: her feet just visible beyond the curtain, jutting out like punctuation in a sentence that wasn't finished. Those same curtains hung between each bed now—not walls, not rooms, just fabric. Thin, striped, stained with the weight of other people's stories.

Standing there again, I recognized what that curtain really was: a veil. A veil that separates this life from whatever waits beyond it. A veil woven with threads of fear and hope, with the hands that have opened and closed it thousands of times. That thin veil witnesses it all—the goodbyes, the prayers, the steadying hands.

One of my patients that day was in isolation, on dialysis, and on a ventilator. He was a large man, silent and still, hidden behind drapes and tubing, bags of nutrients and medications, fluids and filters. No one said, "He can hear you." Not back then. We didn't talk about that. He was reduced to machines and numbers, and I was reduced to tasks.

My task was to help prepare the dialysis fluid. It seemed simple enough—until I missed a medication that needed to be added to one of the bags.

It was a mistake. And in those days, nursing school ran on a three-strikes rule. I had been flawless for two years, but in one moment, I suddenly had two strikes against me.

The instructor that day was not a mentor. Some teachers challenge you to grow. Others challenge your very presence. She was the latter. Her silence stung worse than any reprimand. From then on, I carried her disapproval like a weight strapped to my chest. I walked on eggshells, terrified of another slip—not just of harming a patient, but of being failed out of school for being disliked, not for incompetence.

I didn't fail. I graduated.

But the memory of that experience clung to me.

Weeks later, I walked into my first job in high-risk obstetrics, proud to finally wear the title of nurse. On my first day of orientation, I stepped into the report room—and there she was. The same instructor. Sitting across from me. She didn't look at me. Not once.

I wanted her to see me—really see me. To acknowledge that I had made it. That I was no longer a student, but a peer. But the moment passed in silence. No recognition. No closure.

Looking back, the hardest part of that MICU rotation wasn't the missed medication, though I was horrified. It wasn't even the fear of failing. It was learning how fragile dignity can be in medicine, how quickly a person can be made to feel small.

Years later, I became that nurse. The one who knew her stuff. The one who was fast, precise, in control. Working in high-risk OB, you didn't have the luxury of doubt—when a mother began to bleed or seize, we had five minutes to reach a delivery room and save a life. There's a rush to that kind of nursing.

Knowing your specialty is only half the job. The other half is passing it on.

I see now how that adrenaline can harden you, how certainty can start to sound like superiority. And I became the one I feared in school. Not always. But enough. Enough that matters.

I could have taught more. I could have reached out more. I could have made it easier for the new nurses. And that truth stings.

Because I know what it feels like to be on the other end of it—to be passed over, dismissed, made to feel small by someone who was supposed to help.

Knowing your specialty is only half the job. The other half is passing it on.

The MICU taught me more than how to manage ventilators or dialysis. It taught me how easily fear and shame take root when compassion is absent. It showed me how urgency can harden us if we don't learn to slow down.

I didn't see it then, but this was a glimpse of the patterns that would shape my career: the pull between silence and presence, between performance and compassion. The kind of nurse I would grow into—and eventually, the kind I would have to unlearn to find my way back to myself.

Some curtains mark endings. Others, beginnings. Like my great-aunt Mick, some pass through and return—never to be quite the same. And for those of us still on this side, every step forward changes us, too.

Maybe that's what all beginnings are—crossings of their own. Not just moving forward, but stepping through, changed. Like aunt Mick, I had crossed a threshold too, no longer the same, not yet who I would become.

CHAPTER 6

TOXIC SHOCK

She was my age.

As a brand-new nurse on a gynecology and high-risk obstetrics unit, I wore the fresh white of a new graduate and the invisible weight of someone still waiting to sit for boards. I knew the policy manual like it was scripture and understood just enough to be scared of what I didn't know. One of my first patients was a young woman—my age—admitted with toxic shock syndrome, lupus, and other medical issues. The charts said "guarded." Her face said "tired." Her fever said "now."

I trained that night with an experienced nurse. We did the things we knew to do: hang antibiotics, check labs, chase numbers, cool her down. We slid an aqua-K pad under her—one of those old water-circulating cooling pads they probably don't even make anymore. Her temperature drifted from frightening to manageable, and the room exhaled with us. Small victory, we told ourselves. Maybe the first of many.

Morning shift came. I clocked out. The sun was doing that Iowa thing where it rises like a plain-spoken promise—ordinary, faithful. I drove home believing we had nudged the needle in the right direction.

When I came back the next day, her bed was empty.

I stood in the doorway waiting for a sign that I was in the wrong room—flowers with her name, a blanket folded just so, some proof that she had been moved. I asked the nurse I had been training with what had happened. She didn't look unkind; she looked practiced.

"She died today," she said.

That moment landed hard. I felt a lump rise in my throat, but I swallowed it. I hadn't known she was that sick. I hadn't known she was dying. No one told us. No one told her. There wasn't time—or maybe we didn't know how. We were just trying to bring her fever down.

We were gynecology and high-risk obstetrics. We weren't the ICU, or oncology, or palliative care. We didn't have chaplains rounding or grief carts ready. Death wasn't supposed to come here.

But it did.

And just like before, no one stopped to name what had happened.

The unit kept moving, as it always did. Another patient admitted. Another chart started. The rhythm of care doesn't pause for grief. But something in me had shifted. I went through the motions—med passes, new vitals, the next set of labs—but the silence that followed her stayed with me.

Back then, toxic shock lived for me in a column of symptoms—a sudden storm of infection that could be traced, measured, and treated. It was something you could track in a chart or push back with a timed dose. Sometimes the body turned. Sometimes it didn't.

> ***Toxicity doesn't always come with a fever. It can happen in the body, but also in the spirit, in the heart, in the way we learn to stop feeling so we can keep functioning. Both kinds--physical and emotional--need attention. Both need someone willing to notice.***

Over time I would see toxic shock everywhere—in places that didn't make the textbooks. I saw it in marriages sustained by resentment more than love; in nurses who kept giving until their hands trembled from an emptiness you can't replenish with coffee; in families who held their breath for years because no one would say the hard truth out loud. I saw it in myself when I stayed too long in systems that rewarded speed over soul, perfection over presence. The body always remembers, even when the mouth keeps saying, "I'm fine."

Toxicity doesn't always come with a fever. Sometimes it's quiet. It builds slowly until one day something inside you gives way. It can happen in the body, yes—but also in the spirit, in the heart, in the way we learn to stop feeling so we can keep functioning. Both kinds—physical and emotional—need attention. Both need someone willing to notice.

I didn't have the words for it then, but I have carried the story of this young woman who shared my age for a brief night with me ever since those early nursing days. Her story became a quiet permission slip for me—to tell the truth sooner, to ask the harder questions, to call the chaplain even when the numbers still look "fine."

Her story was one of the first to teach me that life and death often sit side by side, that presence is a kind of medicine, and that even when we can't save, we can still see.

And her story taught me to remember that a human life isn't something you chart; it's someone hoping for another sunrise.

CHAPTER 7

ARIZONA BOUND

One afternoon, after a long night shift, I opened the mailbox and froze.

Inside was a single envelope—thin, ordinary, unremarkable—and yet everything in me knew it carried my future. Back then, if you received a large envelope, it meant you'd passed your nursing boards. A small one meant you hadn't.

I stood on the porch for a long moment, heart pounding, trying to feel the weight of it in my hands, wondering if it was thick enough to hold good news. Finally, I tore it open.

Congratulations.

I had passed.

For a second, I couldn't breathe. Then the tears came. The air itself felt lighter, the world suddenly wider.

For the first time, I felt like I had climbed out from under the weight of every judgement, every doubt, every whispered prediction that a teenage mother couldn't make it.

That afternoon, I waited for Jared to get home from kindergarten. He was five—curious, mischievous, and the center of my world. When he walked through the door, I knelt down and held the letter in front of him like a prize.

"Mommy passed," I said, smiling through tears. "I'm a nurse."

He grinned like it was Christmas morning.

In that moment, I realized it wasn't just my victory—it was ours.

I called my parents next, then my sister and brothers. Their support was every bit a part of the long road to this moment, whether they knew it or not. For the first time, I felt like I had climbed out from under the weight of every judgment, every doubt, every whispered prediction that a teenage mother couldn't make it.

That day at the mailbox, I didn't just become a nurse.

I became someone I could finally be proud of.

I was already a nurse on paper.

Now I needed to become one in my bones.

That knowing didn't arrive all at once.

Life kept moving. I continued working at the University of Iowa. I learned the rhythms of the unit, the weight of responsibility, the muscle memory that only comes with repetition. Jared grew. I settled into the work.

And still, underneath the gratitude and the relief, a quiet question lingered—one I didn't yet know how to answer.

What now?

I had proven I could do it. I could show up for night shifts and early mornings. I could raise a little boy and keep going.

But belonging is different than surviving. Somewhere in that space between the two, something in me began to stir.

And then an old memory surfaced—one that surprised me by how clearly it returned.

I had this dream when I was six years old. I can still see it. I was walking off a plane, the door open behind me, the hum of the engine in the air. In the dream, I wasn't afraid. I was certain. Like I knew I was supposed to step forward.

I hadn't thought about that dream in years. But during that season—after the boards, after the relief, after the *now what?*—it came back to me as if it had been tapped on the shoulder. Not as something mystical. More like a picture that had been waiting quietly its whole life to be remembered.

Looking back, I think the pull had been there all along.

And for reasons I still can't fully explain, when I thought about leaving—about becoming something more than I already was—my mind kept drifting toward the desert.

So I began to look.

Texas came first. I traveled there with my brother Gary—my first real interviews, my first plane ride, my first time learning how to talk about myself as a nurse instead of just surviving shift to shift. Every step felt like stepping into a larger version of myself, even though I didn't yet know what that meant.

But Texas never quite settled in my spirit.

Then came Arizona.

The first time I saw the red rock, I felt my whole body exhale. The mountains looked alive, breathing with color, their edges softened by sunlight. It was June—hot, dry, the kind of heat that wraps around you like an embrace.

I fell in love immediately.

The move itself was equal parts courage and grief.

My sister and I drove to Arizona together—my car packed full, a U-Haul box strapped on top, the rest of my life pared down and purged. What we couldn't carry, we let go of. It felt symbolic, even then.

Leaving my family was the hardest part.

My mom was like a best friend. My dad was always there—steady, protective, quietly making sure Jared and I were okay, helping when we needed it, believing in me even when I doubted myself. We had been through so much together. They had stood with me through the hardest years, and in many ways, they were my reason for striving, growing, and pushing forward.

Walking away from that kind of support wasn't easy. It felt like stepping out without a net.

But I also knew I couldn't stay just because I was safe.

A few months later, I started over in Arizona.

Jared stayed behind for a month and a half while I found my footing. I learned how to get to work, how to find a grocery store, how to make a home. I was terrified and exhilarated all at once—the kind of fear that shows up when you know you're doing something brave.

The first Arizona job felt different—still high-risk obstetrics, but with a pace and scope I'd never seen before. We averaged more than 750 deliveries a month. I worked twelve-hour shifts instead of eight. There were nights I could feel my pulse in the arches of my feet, mornings I'd drive home on autopilot, the desert sun already burning its way up over the horizon.

In Iowa, I had been a new nurse trying to prove myself.

In Arizona, I became a nurse who knew how to survive anything.

Or at least that's what I told myself.

I earned my Clinical Nurse II, then my Clinical Nurse III. Each step meant a raise, more respect, more authority. Dad was proud—money always meant progress to him.

I was proud too.

But behind the credentials, something still just felt hollow.

I loved the work—the precision, the urgency, the privilege of ushering life into the world. But even in those bright delivery rooms, I sometimes felt the old ache return—the silence, the weight, the sense that no matter how many lives we saved, there were losses we still didn't know how to name.

Arizona was a different kind of beautiful—its light sharper, its silence wider. I told myself I'd left Iowa behind, but really, I had only changed the scenery. The habits, the armor, the relentless motion—they all came with me.

Some nights, driving home past the orange glow of the mountains, I'd feel the edges of that old silence stirring again—the one I'd carried since childhood, the one that had followed me through every trauma room and quiet hallway.

But there was something about this place—the open sky, the wide horizons—that began to work on me in ways I couldn't name. The same sun that could burn by day also warmed what had gone cold inside. The landscape held a strange mercy: it didn't demand. It simply waited.

Arizona didn't immediately change me.

But it did begin to soften something—slowly, quietly, insistently.

I may have left Iowa behind, but the stories, the armor, the habits of survival had all hitched a ride.

And here, under a different kind of heat, they began to rise—not to be healed yet, but to be seen.

CHAPTER 8

WHEN LIFE AND DEATH SHARE A BED

Arizona felt like a new beginning—until I realized every beginning carries its own ending.

The desert light poured through the hospital windows, and the mountains stood guard like ancient sentinels. From the outside, my life looked steady. But inside those hospital walls, life and death shared a bed, and I was learning that one always left room for the other.

When I first stepped into the high-risk obstetrics unit, I thought I understood birth.

I'd seen my share of labors in Iowa. I knew the rhythm—the beeps, the charting, the comforting words that sometimes worked and sometimes didn't.

The fetal heart rate monitor gave the baby a voice, an unwavering cadence translated into tones and numbers we trusted to tell us everything was okay.

Or not.

Sometimes there was no fetal voice at all—only the mother's contractions filling the monitor strip, rising and falling like hollow bells. In those moments, the only thing being measured was the labor itself. The absence spoke clearly. What couldn't be tracked or charted often mattered just as much as what could.

But Arizona's pace was its own kind of wild. Babies came faster than we could count—each one a flash of light and sound in the dark hours before dawn. Some nights felt like a current of life surging through the halls; other nights, the silence pressed in around us, heavy and holy, like a held breath.

This was the floor that taught me that every room carried its own story—some beginning, some ending, some doing both at the same time.

It was the floor that taught me that joy and grief have the same address.

One woman I'll never forget labored alone in Room 7. Her contractions were strong, steady, and stubbornly stalled at eight centimeters. I did the usual—checked vitals, monitored contractions—but something felt off. The air in the room was thick, heavy with something unspoken. Finally, I set the chart down and asked quietly, "Is everything okay?"

She hesitated, then whispered, "Today is my mother's birthday. She died a year ago. And now I'm having her first granddaughter."

I understood instantly. Her body was doing what grief does—it was holding on. She hadn't let go yet. I took her hand and said softly, "Your mom will be here. You'll feel her."

Within the hour, she was complete. During delivery, I swear I felt that presence too—the air shifted, softened. Her mother was there. Sometimes a cervix doesn't open because a heart hasn't. That truth changed the way I practiced nursing forever.

Another day, a co-worker was in labor with her first baby. We had pushed for three hours—three hours of sweat, strain, and sheer determination. I wanted so badly for her to have the delivery she hoped for. When the doctor finally called for a C-section, I felt like I had failed her. But she looked at me, calm and smiling, and said,

"It's okay, Leann. The doctor prepared me for this." Her peace caught me off guard. She had already mentally prepared and made peace with having a C-section. I hadn't. That moment stayed with me. Sometimes the lesson isn't about perseverance. It's about release.

Some stories stay with you for decades. Others hide until you're ready to face them. There was a mother who we worked hard to care for her and her baby. The husband and son came to visit every day. On one of those days, the husband and son were in a car accident on their way home from the hospital. They died. I had buried that memory so deep that I didn't even know it was gone until my sister-in-law brought it up years later. "How could you forget that one?" she asked. Her words landed heavy. I had no answer—only the realization that sometimes forgetting is its own form of survival. My heart had made space for so many others, maybe there wasn't room left for that one at the time. But once she reminded me, the memory came rushing back, clear as day. I could see the woman's face, the hospital hallway, the unbearable stillness that followed the news. I wept for her all over again—grief delayed, but not diminished. That story taught me that even when we forget, the body remembers. The soul always knows where the sorrow lies.

Grief is a part of wellness.

A few years later, our hospital participated in a community wellness fair at the mall. Booths lined the walkways, filled with bright posters and healthy slogans—*Prenatal Nutrition*, *Immunizations*, *Safe Sleep for Infants.* Another nurse and I suggested setting up a table for families who had lost a baby—before, during, or shortly after birth.

The administration hesitated. "Why bring death into a wellness fair?" they asked.

"Because grief is part of wellness too," we answered.

That day, women of all ages approached our table with tears in their eyes. They told us about miscarriages they'd never spoken of—one woman shared that hers had happened fifty years earlier, and she had never allowed herself to grieve. Others spoke of babies they'd never been allowed to hold, losses that had been rushed past or silenced.

We handed out brochures, tissues, and gentle acknowledgment. Mostly, we listened. I still remember one woman clutching my hand and saying, *"No one has ever told me it was okay to talk about this."*

Sometimes acknowledgment is the first breath after decades of holding it in. That day, I understood that the need to be seen doesn't expire with time.

A story I will forever carry with me is of the quintuplets—five tiny boys born at just twenty-two weeks. Their parents had refused selective reduction. They couldn't imagine choosing which lives to end. For weeks, the mother lay in bed, feet higher than her head, doing everything she could to hold them.

In the end, her body gave out. I wasn't her nurse during those long weeks, but I was the one who cared for her afterward—and for her husband, whose grief was a storm barely contained.

Later, I went down to the morgue to take pictures of the babies myself—five small, perfect forms wrapped in pink and blue blankets. I didn't do it because I wanted to, but because I knew, even if they couldn't imagine it now, one day they would want to remember.

Years later, I saw her name on the schedule again. She was coming back to deliver a healthy baby. I called to ask if she'd like me there. She didn't hesitate. "Yes, please." When I walked into her room, she smiled through tears. We both knew what it meant to stand together on the other side of loss. I don't know if joy ever truly cancels grief, but sometimes they hold hands and walk together. That day, they did.

Fifteen years in that world. Thousands of mothers. Thousands of stories. So much joy. So much loss.

I thought obstetrics would be about beginnings. But the truth is, every beginning holds an ending. Every cry is shadowed by silence waiting somewhere else down the hall.

CHAPTER 9

BETWEEN TWO WORLDS

This story didn't happen at the beginning of my career, and it didn't happen at the end. It happened somewhere in the middle—before I understood the deeper work I would one day be called to, but after I had already begun to sense that birth and loss often arrive together.

There was a baby who changed the way I saw everything. His name was Michael, and his short life became a compass—one that pointed me toward something I wasn't yet ready for, but somehow had already been prepared to hold.

Birth and death had brushed past each other before in my career, but with Michael, they didn't just pass—they intertwined. His room was the place where I first understood that ushering someone into the world and ushering someone out of it require the same posture: presence, honesty, and a tenderness that asks nothing in return.

Ushering someone into the world and ushering someone out of it require the same posture: presence, honesty, and a tenderness that asks nothing in return.

What happened in those hours with him would stay with me for decades. It would follow me through every shift, every loss, every unraveling. It would echo back to me in moments I didn't yet know were coming.

Some stories stay because they're meant to guide you.

And Michael was one of mine.

It was a busy weekend, the kind where the floor of labor and delivery seemed to breathe on its own—contracting with each new admission, exhaling with each discharge. I had arrived for another twelve-hour shift, the kind that always felt longer when you worked in a unit wired for life. Babies came into the world screaming, pink and furious, and that adrenaline carried us through an entire day.

We were gathered at the desk coordinating assignments when someone mentioned a letter from a neonatologist about a family who would soon arrive to deliver.

"What are you talking about?" I asked, scanning the faces around me.

"There's a letter behind you on the bulletin board."

I turned and saw it immediately—a thick, single-spaced letter pinned at eye level. I slid it from under the pushpin and began to read. It was from a well-known neonatologist, someone whose opinions were never taken lightly. He explained that a family was expecting a baby with anomalies incompatible with life. If the baby didn't die in utero, he would die shortly after birth.

As I read, I felt myself swallowing hard. The words on the page blurred for a moment, their weight settling directly into my chest. Labor and delivery nurses are trained for beginnings, not endings. But sometimes the two arrive holding hands.

When I finished reading, I re-pinned the letter carefully, almost reverently.

A nurse beside me shook her head. "Why in the world are they coming here to deliver? Why not go downtown?"

Her words felt sharp, out of rhythm with the tenderness this family would soon need.

"Probably because this is their community," I said softly. "They want to be close to home and family."

And as I said it, a quiet awareness came over me. *I'll probably be here when this baby is born.* I didn't know how I knew—only that something deep inside me did. A part of me even hoped I would be. Stillbirths and neonatal deaths were the assignments many nurses dreaded. It is just too hard. We're wired for life, especially in labor and delivery.

The weekend passed without that family arriving.

But the next weekend when I returned, little Michael had been born. He was now thirty-six hours old—and still alive.

The unit buzzed with tension. The young couple was exhausted, grieving, and terrified. They didn't know what choices to make. Should they feed him, knowing he likely couldn't digest formula and that surgery wasn't an option? Should they withhold feeding and risk feeling like they caused his suffering? Every path felt wrong. Every decision was heavy with fear and love.

My assignment that day was postpartum. I walked down the hall toward their room with purpose—and, if I'm honest, relief that it was me. I knocked gently, loud enough to be heard, but soft enough that they could choose whether to let me in.

"Please, come in," they said.

Inside, the couple sat quietly, cradling their tiny son. Michael. Perfectly formed on the outside, silently suffering on the inside. The air in the room felt thick, holy—like a place where time moves differently.

I pulled up a chair and sat at their level.

"Can I hold him?" I asked.

They placed him into my arms with the tenderness of people passing their hearts to a stranger and praying I would handle it carefully. His tiny forehead was wrinkled, his breath coming out in gentle, soft grunts—signs we recognize as discomfort. I traced the outline of his little forehead with my finger, memorizing him.

As I cradled him, we talked about the first thirty-six hours of his life, about the impossible choices they had faced, and the X-ray they were waiting on, though everyone knew surgery was not an option. Every decision they made was based in love, even when none of the choices felt like mercy.

"You're doing the right things," I reassured them. "You're doing what feels right for *your* baby."

Just then, the portable X-ray machine barreled loudly down the hallway, rattling against the doorframe. The jarring sound collided with the sacred quiet of the moment. I held up my hand in a gentle stop.

"Can you come back later?" I asked the technician, my voice soft but protective.

And then I spoke to Michael, my voice a whisper meant for both him and his parents.

"Babies aren't supposed to die," I said.

His father, eyes red and stunned, looked at me and said, "Maybe they are, Leann."

His words hung between us—raw, unfiltered truth. Sometimes love requires witnessing a pain that cannot be fixed. Sometimes presence is the only medicine left.

The four of us sat quietly. The threshold between life and death felt so close, like Michael was balanced right at its edge.

Gently, I asked, "Have you told Michael it's okay to die?"

They stared at me, startled. "Are we supposed to do that?" the father asked.

"I don't know," I said honestly. "But you'll know if you need to."

There was something about that moment—something instinctive, almost ancient.

It wasn't medical.

It wasn't procedural.

It was midwifing a letting-go, the same way we midwife a letting-in.

I handed Michael back to his mother and told them to call if they needed anything.

Forty-five minutes later, the hallway light outside their room went off.

I walked in.

Michael had died—peacefully, in his parents' arms.

"Would you like me to listen for a heartbeat?" I asked quietly.

"You can if you need to, Leann," his father said. "Whatever you need to do."

I stepped out and called the pediatrician, who had been expecting this moment.

"The baby died," I said.

"What happened?"

"They gave him permission," I answered. "And he was able to die."

Silence filled the line. The truth didn't need more words.

Later that morning, the family was ready to go home, to step into a world that no longer held their son. As I helped them into their car, they turned to me with tears in their eyes.

"Thank you," they said. "For what you do. For who you are."

"You're very welcome," I told them.

And then I pushed the empty wheelchair back toward labor and delivery. It felt heavier than it should have, as though the weight of the morning had settled into its frame. Waiting at the elevator, grief washed over me—not just sadness for the family, but tenderness, gratitude, awe.

Michael had been born into this world and left it in the same room, in the same arms. He taught me that witnessing is sacred work. That presence can usher in peace. That sometimes the most faithful act we can offer is neither to intervene nor to turn away—but simply to stay.

Witnessing is sacred work. Sometimes the most faithful act we can offer is neither to intervene nor turn away--but simply to stay.

As the elevator doors closed, I felt it settle in my bones: Babies aren't supposed to die.

But some do. And when they do, someone has to sit beside them at the threshold.

Someone has to hold the space between two worlds.

CHAPTER 10

CROSSING THE THRESHOLD

For fifteen years, labor and delivery had shaped me—steady rhythms, predictable protocols, a world where beginnings were the language we spoke. I had grown into that identity the way a body grows into a uniform: familiar, expected, almost second skin. But somewhere deep inside, a tightness had begun to form. A quiet pressure. A sense that the work I knew so well was no longer the full measure of who I was becoming.

I couldn't name it yet. I only knew something in me was straining, stretching—pushing against edges I hadn't realized were there.

And then came the week everything shifted.

The day we lost our first pregnant mother I felt the ground shift beneath me. She'd written in her journal that she knew she was going to die, that she just wanted to see her baby. She did. And then she was gone. Two more mothers followed in quick succession—one from fatty liver disease, another unexpectedly. Three deaths in such a short span.

After the third, I found myself in the stairwell between floors, trembling, whispering a prayer I didn't even know I knew.

"Lord, I need a break."

I thought I was asking for rest. What I didn't know was that I was asking for transformation.

That transformation didn't come all at once.

Instead, I stepped away from the hospital and into a very different season of work—leaving the bedside to join a large OB/GYN group as a director of marketing. I moved fast, stayed busy, and felt important again. On the outside, it looked like success. On the inside, it was momentum without stillness. I was living in the fast lane, telling myself I was fine.

It would take time—and more unraveling—before the road narrowed and hospice began to call.

Eventually, hospice began showing up everywhere I turned. A commercial on television while I drank my morning coffee. An article in the paper about a new hospice house opening in town. A help-wanted ad tucked in the corner of a newsletter that somehow made its way to my desk.

Each time, I brushed it off. *Coincidence,* I told myself. "I'm a labor nurse," I'd say out loud. "Not a death nurse."

But something deeper knew the truth. Part of me was loosening its grip on the nurse I had been, making room for the nurse I was becoming.

A few months later, I accepted a position in hospice admissions. The transition was jarring. After fifteen years of welcoming life, I was now walking with people as they prepared to leave it.

I remember sitting in a training session when the bereavement coordinator turned to me and said, "Leann, you have to say it. Say it three times: *when you die, die, die.*"

I couldn't do it. The words lodged in my throat.

In obstetrics, we never said death out loud—it was the unspoken thing. But in hospice, it had to be named, faced, honored. That day, I realized how far I still had to go. Saying the word felt like crossing a threshold, one I'd been circling my entire career without realizing it.

Every labor, every loss, every whispered prayer in the stillness of a hospital room was doing its quiet work. Together, they were teaching me how to sit with the sacred—how to be fully present in the space between holding on and letting go.

> *Every labor, every loss, every whispered prayer in the stillness of a hospital room was doing its quiet work. They were teaching me how to sit with the sacred—how to be fully present in the space between holding on and letting go.*

A seam had opened inside of me, and the work I had once fit so easily into no longer felt like it could hold me.

All those years, I'd been midwifing the beginning of life. Now, I was being called to midwife its end.

CHAPTER 11

THE SMALLEST BONE

When I first prayed for a break, I didn't expect God to take me so literally.

I had meant rest—a weekend off, maybe a lighter schedule. What I got instead was stillness of an entirely different kind.

By now, hospice had become familiar—its rhythms, its stillness, the sacred quiet of rooms where last breaths were taken with tenderness. I had gone from being the nurse who welcomed life to the one who walked with people as they prepared to leave it. The work was holy, but it was heavy, too. And somewhere along the way, I began to fill every empty space in my life with motion.

I didn't see it happening at first. That's how slow unravelings usually begin.

Time passed. Jared grew older. My role expanded. I was good at what I did, and the healthcare world took notice. Eventually I moved into leadership—managing programs, building teams, sitting in meetings that stretched long past lunch. I told myself it was growth. I told myself it was purpose. But the truth was simpler: I didn't know how to stop moving.

Hospice work had taught me to sit with the dying, but I still didn't know how to sit with myself.

I woke before dawn to answer demands that never slept. I worked through lunch. I carried grief in one pocket and urgency in the other, both buzzing with needs that felt endless. I told myself this was success, but it was really survival with a shinier name.

Jared saw the truth before I did.

One evening, as I rushed through the kitchen—purse in hand, thoughts two days ahead—he looked up from his homework and asked, almost gently, "Why are you always in such a hurry, Mom?"

I laughed it off, offered something half-true, and kept moving. But his question followed me down every hallway, into every meeting, even into the hospice rooms where I told families to breathe while I forgot to do it myself.

Somewhere in this season, our office sponsored a softball team. I agreed to play because I thought I needed more "fun."

I penciled it in like another task.

It was late in the game when it happened.

Dust rising. Laughter somewhere behind me. Then a slide into third base, gravel biting into my palms—and a tiny, unmistakable *snap.* A sound too small for what it changed.

At first I thought it was nothing. I even tried to stand. But my ankle buckled, pain radiating upward like fire. By the next morning it had swollen to twice its size.

The orthopedic surgeon barely looked at me.

"Maybe what you need," he said, scribbling on a pad, "is an antidepressant."

His words stunned me. I wanted to say, *You don't even know me.* I wasn't depressed; I was depleted. I wasn't broken; I was disconnected. I didn't argue, but I didn't accept the prescription either. I thanked him and hobbled out on crutches, carrying something heavier than pain—an ache of not being seen.

It was a familiar ache. In time, it would become useful.

For the first time in decades, I couldn't go anywhere.

No twelve-hour shifts. No late-night emails. No multi-tasking my way through exhaustion. Just stillness—me, my cast, and the long quiet days that followed.

At first the silence was unbearable. Then it became its own kind of medicine.

Jared was in high school by then. He helped with small things—groceries, laundry, reminders to elevate my leg. We ate dinner at the table again. Talked. Laughed. Sometimes we just sat together watching the desert light change on the walls.

Somewhere in the middle of those days, I did something I wasn't used to doing. I called my mom and asked for help.

I didn't have a clear plan or a list—I only knew that I needed her.

There was a pause. Then she said, "You have never asked for help." Within days, she was on a plane. That was my mom—dependable strength, whatever life asked of her.

I began to realize the pain wasn't just in my ankle. It lived in every part of me I had ignored—muscles tight with striving, breath shallow from years of rushing, heart heavy with unspoken grief.

One afternoon in a bookstore, a title seemed to reach for me: *Full Catastrophe Living* by Jon Kabat-Zinn. The title made me laugh—it felt too on the nose—but I started reading. His words landed like truth I had always known but never practiced: that healing isn't about doing more, it's about learning to be present; that pain is not the enemy, but a messenger.

So I began to listen—to my breath, to my body, to the ache behind the hurry. Each day, the noise inside me softened just a little.

I'd spent most of my life running—toward goals, away from feelings, into every crisis that needed fixing. But the fracture forced me to stop. It made me face what I'd been outrunning: myself.

Sometimes I think the body knows long before the soul catches up.

Mine had been whispering for years—through fatigue, headaches, the hollow ache that followed even my proudest moments. I just hadn't been listening.

Now, immobilized, I finally heard it.

It was the smallest bone that finally cracked the hardest truth—*I couldn't heal others until I learned to stop and listen to myself.*

I couldn't heal others until I learned to stop and listen to myself.

That break marked the end of one life and the quiet beginning of another.

The undoing had already begun.

PART II

THE UNDOING

The cocoon closes around her, and the quiet becomes deeper still. In the dark, what she was begins to loosen—softened by grace, reshaped by something she can't yet name.

INTERLUDE

THE KNOWINGS

Before the undoing came the *knowings.*

They didn't shout; they whispered. A nudge in my chest when I ignored what I felt. A heaviness in my stomach when I said yes but meant no.

For years I called it stress, or exhaustion, or just the cost of caring. But the body remembers what the mind can't yet name. It tells the truth in tension, in restlessness, in the quiet ache that begs you to stop running.

The unraveling had begun. The same stillness I'd feared all my life was calling me closer—not to break me apart, but to show me what had been speaking inside me all along.

CHAPTER 12

WHEN EVERYTHING CHANGED

Jared's question came back to haunt me during those long, motionless weeks.

"Mom, why are you always in a hurry?"

At the time, I'd brushed it off. But now—sitting on the couch, my ankle wrapped, my calendar blank for the first time in years—it echoed in my mind. *Do I ever slow down?* And even more haunting: *Why don't I?*

The ankle injury became an invitation.

An invitation to rest.
To listen.
To stop measuring my worth by motion.

Stillness felt foreign at first. I'd been so used to rushing through my days—solving, fixing, producing—that silence felt like failure. But when the noise stopped, I began to notice the ache beneath it all. The exhaustion wasn't just physical; it was spiritual.

I started to think about the people I'd cared for over the years—the patients I'd hurried through, the ones whose stories I hadn't taken time to hear. I understood now, in a way I never could before that visit with the orthopedic doctor, what it felt like to be unseen. I'd spent years treating bodies while quietly neglecting my own. The irony wasn't lost on me.

That forced stop stripped away everything unnecessary. And in that emptiness, something holy began to stir.

When my job ended not long after, I didn't fall apart the way I might have once. The fear was still there, but underneath it was a strange calm—as if some deeper part of me already knew this was how change begins.

Weeks into my unplanned pause, I saw in the newspaper: Holistic Nurse Wanted—Healing Center, Sedona.

The words glowed on the page. I didn't even know what "holistic nursing" meant, but something in me leaned forward. I called, applied, interviewed, and within weeks, I was on my way to train with the Gerson Institute in San Marcos, California.

Our instructor, Charlotte Gerson, was fierce and brilliant—uncompromising in her belief that the body knows how to heal when given the chance. She taught us that healing wasn't a war we fought, but a rhythm we joined.

In traditional medicine, healing meant medications, interventions, charting, and stabilizing. It meant assigning numbers to symptoms, documenting progress, and staying two steps ahead of whatever might go wrong. Here in California where my Gerson training began, healing looked nothing like that.

We woke before dawn to prepare fresh juices from nearly twenty pounds of produce each day—carrot juice, green juice, carrot-apple. We learned how food carried its own kind of intelligence, how nutrients could do what pharmaceuticals sometimes couldn't.

Instead of pain medications, we used clay packs, castor oil packs, and coffee enemas—tools I had been taught to dismiss as strange or outdated, yet I watched them reduce pain faster than anything in my medicine cart ever had.

We learned to observe skin tone, breath, posture, and the tone of a patient's voice—not as subjective impressions, but as meaningful clinical information.

I was used to care plans. Options. Protocols.

Here, the work required something different—presence, instinct, curiosity, reverence.

Traditional nursing had taught me to assess the body.

This work was teaching me to *listen* to it.

And the biggest surprise of all: I was required to go through every part of the therapy myself before I could offer it to anyone else. That meant stripping my body of things I had never questioned—no makeup, no nail polish, no antiperspirant, no perfume, no lipstick. Everything that masked, scented, or sealed the body was considered toxic. I had to meet myself bare, without the small protections I'd worn for years.

It was humbling, even brutal at times. My body protested at first—nausea, headaches, tears. But beneath the discomfort, I could feel something shifting. Something that wasn't just physical. A quiet knowing. A whisper of *Pay attention. Something is changing.*

From California, we traveled to Hospital Meridian in Tijuana, Mexico—a quiet, concrete place where patients came seeking last chances. The air was heavy with hope and fear.

That's where I met her—the young woman with no hair. She was sitting in the cafeteria, eyes soft and clear. I froze. Something in me recognized her, though we'd never met. I turned to Charlotte and whispered, "Tell me I can do this."

She smiled. "You can do this."

Later, I sat beside the young woman. She studied my face for a long moment before asking, "Why are you doing this?"

"I don't know," I said honestly. "I just know I'm supposed to be here. It feels right."

She nodded, as if that was enough.

"You can beat this," I said. And I meant it—not as a promise of outcome, but as a declaration of presence.

That trip marked the beginning of my undoing. I had come to learn how to help others heal. Instead, I was learning how to *see.*

When I finally arrived at the Gerson Healing Center in Sedona, the desert itself felt alive—its red rocks like open palms catching the light. I'd seen beauty before, but not like this. Sedona pulsed with something ancient, something that asked for reverence.

The work there was relentless and sacred. We rose before dawn, blending and juicing for hours. Patients arrived from around the world—some skeptical, some desperate, all of them searching for hope.

This work never felt like hospice to me, even though many of our patients had already been through it all—surgery, radiation, chemotherapy—once, twice, sometimes three times. They didn't come to us because we were the first option. They came because someone had told them, "There's nothing more we can do."

We were not their saviors. We were companions. Witnesses.

Each patient carried a story, and each story carried its own kind of holiness.

Emily was one of my first patients. I still see her face when I think about Sedona.

She arrived just before dusk, walking slowly beside her husband, Kyle. He hovered the way a man does when he's terrified of losing the one person he doesn't know how to live without. They were polite, grateful, trying hard to be hopeful—but underneath, something felt tight. Fragile. Emily had rectal cancer.

That first night, Kyle followed her every move. He carried her bags, tucked her blankets, watched every expression that crossed her face. He asked questions before she could answer them. He wanted so badly to fix what he couldn't fix. To protect her from something no one could protect her from.

I saw in him what I've seen in many spouses: fear that had become control, and control that looked like love. It wasn't abusive. It wasn't intentional. It was survival.

When Emily couldn't sleep that first night, she padded into the hall asking for Tylenol—something we didn't offer there. She looked almost apologetic for needing anything. "I don't want to bother anyone," she whispered.

But her eyes were pleading for more than a pain reliever. There was a heaviness around her that didn't feel physical. Later, I told one of the doctors how unsettled I felt. "I don't know what it is," I said, "but something is sitting on her chest besides the cancer."

The doctor looked at me and said gently, "Then ask her. That's your job here."

After the shift change, I went into her room, sat on the floor, and looked up at her. She sat stiffly in her chair, hands folded, as if bracing herself for bad news.

"Emily," I said softly, "I don't think your body can heal until something inside you loosens. I don't know what it is, but I think *you* probably do."

For a long moment, she stared at her hands. Then her chin trembled. Then the truth rose.

"It's him," she said quietly.

Not sharply. Not angrily. Just honestly. She pointed toward the door—not at a villain, but at a man she had lived beside for decades.

"He's peeled and poked away at me for so many years," she said. "He doesn't do it to be cruel. He's scared. But I can't breathe around his fear anymore. I'm tired, Leann."

Her words were not an accusation. They were a *release.*

A naming. A letting out. The first breath she had taken in a very long time.

We talked about what it meant to finally tell the truth—not to blame, but to unburden. To separate his fear from her responsibility. To give herself permission to heal without carrying both their anxieties on her back.

She didn't ask for advice. She just needed someone to hear her. When I left the room that night, she looked lighter. Not cured—but clearer.

I didn't know what would happen the next morning. I worried that Kyle would be hurt or angry or confused. I worried Emily might retreat, apologize, and take it all back.

Instead, Kyle found me at the nursing desk. "Leann," he said, voice shaky, "I need to tell you something." My stomach dropped.

But then he took my hand. "Thank you," he said, eyes full. "Thank you for whatever you said to Emily. You saw something we couldn't name. You've changed our lives."

And that's when I understood: It wasn't about him being the problem. It was about her finally being allowed to tell the truth. And about him being willing to hear it.

That moment didn't just shift Emily's healing. It shifted their marriage.

And it shifted me.

Because I learned that healing isn't always about tumors shrinking or lab values normalizing.

Sometimes healing begins with one brave sentence: "This is what's hurting me."

Sometimes that's the medicine the body has been waiting for.

Our second patient, Lorna, was impossible to miss—a vibrant redhead who filled the hallway before she ever introduced herself. She looked me over with a mischievous grin and said, "Are you a patient or a nurse? Hard to tell around here."

She had been through more than most bodies can endure: multiple biopsies, colon removal, metastases to the liver. Her first oncologist had given her six years without looking her in the eye.

"I'll go to *his* funeral one day," she joked.

That was Lorna—fire, humor, and defiance braided together.

That night I sat on the floor of her room while she unpacked her story. Unlike Emily, she didn't hesitate.

"I'm tired of being treated like a diagnosis," she said. "I'm still me."

And she was.

She jogged to the dining room to play the organ. She joked with the new arrivals while wearing clay packs wrapped dramatically around her head. She laughed so hard she cried, and then cried so hard she laughed again.

She taught me that emotion isn't messy—it's honest. It's what moves. It's what heals.

Paula was quieter. Still.

She had a way of looking at me like she could see beneath the surface. "I feel a presence when you walk into the room," she whispered once.

Her words unnerved me because they were true. Something in me was expanding—intuition, awareness, sensitivity—things traditional nursing had trained out of me.

But here, they were required.

Honored.

Needed.

Then came Howard—a young father, already hollowed by two brain surgeries, walking in with his wife and their five-week-old baby. That tiny infant felt like a prayer carried through the doorway.

His wife's sadness filled the room before her words did. Fear sat between them like a third presence, but so did love—raw, desperate, luminous. Some nights I prayed for them on my drive home, my hands tight on the steering wheel.

Howard taught me how much courage it takes to stay soft when life has been unbearably hard.

Ernie arrived with lymphoma and a weariness that had been mistaken for hopelessness. But his body responded immediately—shockingly—to the therapy. His tumors visibly shrank. You could see the changes with the naked eye.

Watching him was like watching the body remember how to heal. It undid something in me—this quiet truth that sometimes the body knows long before we do.

Not every patient came with fire or fight. Some arrived already half in this world and half in the next.

One night I sat with Mary, a woman who was very sick and very tired—too tired to pretend she wasn't afraid.

"I don't want to fight anymore," she whispered.

Her words weren't surrender. They were honesty—pure, unfiltered, holy honesty.

As we talked, she reached toward my chest and took hold of the necklace I always wore—a tiny stork charm from my years catching babies in labor and delivery. She held it gently between her fingers.

Her eyes softened the way someone's eyes do when they are speaking from the edge of two worlds. "Leann," she said, "you're birthing people at an entirely different level now."

Her words didn't land on me—they settled *in* me.

And just like that, my two worlds—birth and death—were no longer separate. I was still a midwife. Only now, I was midwifing a different kind of passage.

And she, without knowing it, midwifed something in me, too.

Not every story ended with recovery. Like Mary, some of our patients died. But even those endings carried meaning. Healing, I was learning, doesn't always mean surviving. Sometimes it means surrendering with grace.

The longer I worked there, the more I noticed things I couldn't explain—the warmth in my hands when I prayed with someone, the calm that filled a room when fear finally loosened its grip. There were moments when I wanted to jump out of my skin and run out the door, especially when the unknown pressed too close. These were things I had never been grounded in before—things I had never even believed could happen. And that was frightening, because it forced me to confront a truth that many people avoid: the spiritual dimension of life. The part no one talks about. The part that gets you labeled as "crazy" if you dare speak it out loud.

But instead of running, I stayed.

Sedona taught me that healing isn't about doing—it's about *being*. It's about the stillness that makes space for something larger to move through us.

> ***Healing isn't about doing—it's about* being. *It's about the stillness that makes space for something larger to move through us.***

We worked hard, we cried often, and we laughed whenever we could. But beneath it all, I began to feel a gentle unraveling inside myself. I was learning to release the armor that had held me together for so long—the need to prove, to perform, to control outcomes.

It was a beautiful undoing.

Contrary to everything I had learned up to that point in my training and career, I discovered that healing isn't always about curing. Sometimes it's about witnessing. Holding space. Walking someone to the threshold. Helping them find their voice—or their breath—one last time.

I came to understand the look in someone's eyes when they're no longer fully here. I became fluent in a new kind of silence. Comfortable with presence. Open to mystery.

This was more than medicine.
This was soul work.

Still, I was exhausted. My body, always the truth-teller, began to whisper again—this time through fatigue, tension, and small symptoms I didn't want to name. I brushed them off, the way I always had.

Then came the test results: Abnormal cells. Repeat testing. Procedures. Words like *dysplasia* and *precancerous.*

For the first time, I wasn't the nurse. I was the patient.

I remember sitting in my car outside the clinic, staring at the steering wheel, whispering into the quiet: "Okay, God. I'm listening."

It struck me then—my patients had been teaching me something long before my body forced me to learn it.

Truth-telling is healing.
Letting go is healing.
Slowing down is healing.
Seeing yourself is healing.

Sedona had taught me what healing looked like in others. Everything I had watched unfold in them—the courage, the surrender, the honesty, the presence—was now the work I had to do inside myself.

Their stories had been the beginning of my undoing.

This diagnosis would be the continuation of it.

Now, it was time to live it myself.

CHAPTER 13

MY HEALING JOURNEY

I didn't know I was entering a cocoon when I began working at the Gerson Healing Center in Sedona, Arizona. I thought I was simply stepping into a new job. A beautiful one. A place where prevention, nourishment, and holistic care surrounded every patient—and now, finally, surrounded me too.

About sixty days in, something inside me began to slow down. Not my work. Not my schedule. Me.

It began so simply, with routine self-care—something nurses are notoriously bad at. I scheduled my first mammogram. I got new glasses and contacts. I went to the dentist and made plans to remove my mercury fillings. I completed my annual pap smear.

Normal things. Responsible things.

And then everything shifted.

When my pap smear came back abnormal, my first reaction wasn't fear. It was panic—the kind that rises fast and makes you feel small inside your own body.

I brought my chart to a provider I had trusted for years. She reassured me kindly and professionally, saying we'd just repeat the test in three months. So we did.

The results came back the same.

This time, my worry rooted itself deeply.

I needed a colposcopy. I remember sitting in the office as the provider tried to soothe me with statistics, saying I had a greater chance of being hit by a car than having something serious show up in the biopsy.

Her attempt at reassurance felt cold, detached—a math equation in place of empathy. Instead of comforting me, it made me feel profoundly unseen. Unheard. As if fear needed to be talked out of me rather than tended to.

That was the moment the cocoon began to wrap itself around me—quietly, tightly, without permission.

The colposcopy confirmed severe dysplasia. A step before cancer. A whisper from my own body that something wasn't okay.

I received the news while standing in the energetic heart of the Gerson Healing Center—a place where prayers, tears, and hope coexisted under the same roof.

Dr. Melendez, one of our consultants from Mexico, took my hands and prayed. She told me she had been through the same thing thirty-five years earlier. She was calm. Centered. Certain. She reminded me that thoughts carry power—and that I didn't have to rush the next step.

But even her reassurance couldn't fully quiet the fear.

I opened up to a few staff members, letting myself be held for once instead of being the one holding others. Their support steadied me, but the truth was still heavy: This wasn't someone else's crisis.

This was mine.

The physician performing the procedure was my former boss—someone I had worked with for nearly a decade. A man whose steadiness had helped shape my early nursing years. As he explained each step, his eyes filled with tears.

"You know I'm not going to let anything happen to you, don't you LeLe?" he said.

I nodded, crying too.

His compassion cracked something open in me. For years I had been the strong one, the steady one, the one families and patients leaned on. But here, in this sterile room under bright lights, I was the one who needed holding.

It felt unfamiliar. And holy.

When I first received the biopsy results, I remember asking a coworker, "Why is this happening?"

Everyone had an answer. The one I heard most often was that maybe the Creator wanted me to understand firsthand what patients go through. Maybe this was meant to deepen my empathy, to teach me what couldn't be taught any other way.

Their words were well-intentioned and maybe partly true. But it also felt like it had gone a step too far. This wasn't a lesson. This was my body. My health. My life. And for the first time, I realized how fragile everything truly is. How quickly life can tilt. How little control I actually have.

It was humbling. It was terrifying. And it made one truth impossible to ignore: I could not keep pouring from an empty cup.

The options laid out before me felt overwhelming—a LEEP (Loop Electrosurgical Excision Procedure), cone biopsy, or hysterectomy. That last word hit me like a stone. Hysterectomy. It felt final. Extreme. Too much for my age. Too much to process.

So I agreed to the LEEP. I had the procedure. And then—I went to work that same night. No rest. No pause. No gentle permission to tend to my own healing. Just the old pattern: push through, show up, keep moving.

Inside the cocoon, old habits don't break all at once. They soften, melt, and slowly stop fitting the shape of who you're becoming.

The Healing Center became a kind of sanctuary. Staff members hugged me and prayed over me. The building itself seemed to hum with mercy.

And in the quiet moments, I finally allowed myself to admit what I had ignored for too long: I was tired. I was scared. I wasn't dealing with everything. I felt fragile—like a little girl standing alone in a big, unpredictable world.

One afternoon, in the stillness of a treatment room, I heard it clearly—not audibly, but unmistakably: *What are you really afraid of, Leann?*

The question wasn't harsh. It wasn't shaming. It was gentle, curious, inviting. It felt like the first crack in the cocoon. Not the part where you break out—not yet. Just the part where you stop fighting the transformation you didn't choose.

My healing didn't begin with the procedure or the prayers or the statistics or even the fear.

My healing began when I realized that I couldn't keep caring for others while abandoning myself.

It began the moment I listened.

The moment I acknowledged that something had to change. That I couldn't keep caring for others while abandoning myself. That healing wasn't something I gave—it was something I needed.

Inside the cocoon, everything softens before it becomes. Everything dissolves before it takes shape.

In that sacred, trembling space between fear and faith, I began to heal—from the inside out.

CHAPTER 14

MEETING ELISABETH KÜBLER-ROSS

Long before Sedona, long before the unraveling that would reshape my life, there was a classroom moment from a course on death and dying I assumed had passed me by—a name I didn't expect to follow me beyond the exam.

Elisabeth Kübler-Ross.

Years later, her name surfaced again. Not in a classroom this time, but in the foyer of a silent auction for a local hospice—an event filled with artwork and soft conversation. I wasn't expecting anything meaningful to happen there. I certainly wasn't expecting my life to turn.

But then I saw it: a framed photograph of Elisabeth Kübler-Ross and Mother Teresa.

Something inside me stirred. I couldn't explain it. I placed a bid and lingered nearby, wanting to keep an eye on the bidding sheet.

As the program began, a door on the far side of the room suddenly opened, and a woman in a wheelchair was pushed through. It was her.

Elisabeth Kübler-Ross.

In the flesh.

The woman whose words had lingered in the back of my mind for years.

Before my mind caught up, my feet were already moving toward her. I reached out to shake her hand. She immediately pulled back. "Don't touch," she said. "People with cancer have enormous pain."

But then she extended her index finger for an "E.T. touch." Finger to finger. It was a greeting without hurt. A boundary delivered with kindness.

I told her I had bid on the photograph of her and Mother Teresa and asked if she would sign it if I won. Before she could respond, the woman pushing her wheelchair said, "You can call her. She's in the phone book," and whisked her away.

I remember thinking, *As if Elisabeth Kübler-Ross is in the phone book.*

But the idea wouldn't leave me.

I waited a week before searching. Back then, the Arizona phone book was enormous—an encyclopedia of names. I flipped through page after page until I saw it: Kübler-Ross, Elisabeth. I stared at the entry, then dialed.

She answered.

I said, "I bid on the photo of you and Mother Teresa, and although I didn't get it . . . can I come visit you?"

"Yes," she said easily.

She gave me her address, told me the door would be unlocked, and said, "Come in when you arrive."

Her home sat deep in the desert—dirt roads, long stretches of quiet, hand-painted wooden signs with arrows pointing to *Elisabeth*. A tepee stood in the yard. A tall totem pole watched the sky.

The front door, heavy and wooden like the morgue door I once feared, was unlocked just as she promised. Inside, she sat in her recliner across the room, television blaring, a tray full of empty cups beside her.

"Did you find it alright?" she asked.

I laughed. "I knew I had the right house when I saw the tepee."

She smiled, held out her finger for the E.T. touch, and pointed to the couch overflowing with manuscripts. "Sit."

I perched on a small corner.

"Have you read *The Wheel of Life*?" she asked. This was one of the books Elisabeth had written.

"Not yet."

She pointed toward the door.
"Go read it. Come back after you do."

It wasn't harsh. It was honest. If I wanted to engage with her, I needed to understand her work.

I left, bought the book, read it, and returned.

I came back two weeks later, knocking lightly even though she had said the door would be unlocked. It felt strange to enter the home of someone so well-known simply by walking in.

The moment I stepped inside, she didn't waste a second.

"Go in the refrigerator," she said, "get the bean soup. Heat it up and bring me a big spoon."

So there I was again—standing in Elisabeth Kübler-Ross's kitchen, heating her lunch, feeling both honored and slightly stunned by the ordinariness of it. When the soup was warm, I carried it back to her along with a paper towel.

She had a pillow on her lap. I placed the paper towel gently on top of it.

"Pick that up," she said, "it's too heavy."

I blinked. *The paper towel?* But I lifted it back up and watched as she laid a single Kleenex on the pillow instead.

"That's not as heavy," she said, and nodded toward the soup. "Put it in a smaller, lighter cup."

When she asked me to remove the paper towel because it was "too heavy," I realized how much pain she lived with. Not the kind you chart or medicate, but the kind that shapes every small movement. A single sheet of Kleenex was all her body could tolerate. That moment stayed with me—a reminder that real suffering is often silent and easily overlooked.

> ***Real suffering is often silent and easily overlooked.***

I sat on the corner of the couch—barely enough room between stacks of manuscripts—and words spilled out of me fast. Too fast. I told her about my dream of opening a hospice and healing center. About Sedona. About the Gerson Healing Center. About the patients who came after selling their homes and horses and everything they owned for one last hope.

She listened while eating her soup, her eyes sharp, unwavering.

"You work for a for-profit hospice?" she asked.

"Yes."

She shook her head. "Not-for-profit is the only way to go," she said, as if it were simply fact.

I nodded, still chattering, until she cut through my rambling with a single sentence that stopped me cold.

"First you must get rid of your junk."

I blinked. "My what?"

"Your baggage," she said firmly. "You cannot help other people until you deal with your own."

It felt random but also perfect because I knew she was right. I just didn't know how to start.

"You need to go see Joseph," she said. "He's my healer. As far as I'm concerned, he's the only good one. The rest are fakes." She recited his phone number from memory.

"He charges $100," she added, "but he's worth $10,000."

We talked more about Sedona—about the patients who came desperate for healing, about the ones who did well and the many who didn't. She asked questions no one else ever had—not clinical questions, but soulful ones.

I was scribbling notes as quickly as I could when she stopped eating and stared at me.

"Why are you writing all this down?"

"Because I don't want to forget," I said.

She smiled and shook her head as if amused that I thought I could capture everything she was giving me on a piece of paper.

Birds were flocking outside her window, loud and insistent. I kept turning to watch them—she noticed and didn't mind. They were part of the atmosphere around her, as if they, too, had something to say.

I asked if she ever got lonely.

"No," she said. "Two people visit every day. One in the morning and one in the afternoon."

"Are you able to get around?" I asked.

"I have no choice," she said, lighting a cigarette. The smoke drifted softly around her face, giving her an almost timeless look—wise, worn, and utterly present. She seemed both grounded in her body and far beyond it at the same time, as if she lived in two worlds at once.

"Look at yourself first," she said, suddenly serious. "Get rid of your unfinished business."

"How will I know when I've done that?" I asked.

"When you don't react negatively to anything anymore," she answered, as if that were the simplest thing in the world.

She told me to read *Working It Through* and then come back.

Three weeks later, I arrived for my third visit with chocolates and lavender oil. As I approached her yard, I saw them—hawks. Six of them, perched on her totem pole, loud and fierce, commanding the sky. I took pictures, stunned by the scene.

Inside, she greeted me with her widest smile yet and held out her finger for the E.T. hello.

We talked about her book. "I haven't read any of my twenty-six," she laughed.

I shared the lines that stayed with me—about God giving us what we need, about curative power beyond medicine, about patients longing for honesty and peace, and how sometimes the right response is simply taking a breath when you don't know what to say.

She listened, amused and tender, as if seeing her work through fresh eyes.

I asked if it got easier after forty years.

"It doesn't matter," she said simply.

Then she leaned forward, as if moving from reflection into instruction.

Her tone shifted. She explained that professional denial often keeps patients from sharing their deepest concerns.

Then she made it personal. About my dream of opening a healing center, she said the place wasn't important—it was the work that mattered.

She talked about learning self-love and forgiveness so that I could one day offer those gifts to others.

When I admitted I hadn't seen Joseph yet because of money, her expression sharpened.

"His visit is the most important," she said firmly. "The most."

As she grew tired, she leaned back against her chair.

Then the phone rang. She glanced at the caller ID and gave me a soft, knowing smile.

"Joseph," she said, lifting the receiver.

I stood to leave and offered the E.T. goodbye. She extended her finger without missing a beat, still talking to him as I slipped out the door.

Outside, the desert was quiet. The hawks were gone. Only stillness remained.

Later I would learn that in ancient Egypt, the hawk symbolized the soul—swift, watchful, a messenger inviting you to see from a higher perspective. At the time, I didn't know any of that. I only knew that six hawks had greeted me when I arrived, and now not one remained.

It felt like a sign—not that something outside of me had shifted, but that something *inside* me had.

Their absence told me what their presence couldn't: the message had already been delivered. The awakening was already happening within me.

I stood there a moment longer, letting the stillness rest softly over me.

Not an ending.
A beginning.

CHAPTER 15

BIRTH AND DEATH ARE THE SAME THING

Meeting Elisabeth had stirred something in me, but the teaching that followed began to rearrange me from the inside out. It wasn't like school—no lectures, no textbooks, no outlines. Her lessons came in the form of conversations, gestures, pauses, and everyday tasks that somehow held the weight of ceremony.

During one visit, I sat across from her and told her the simplest truth about myself. "I'm a nurse," I said. "I've worked from birth to death—labor and delivery and now hospice."

She didn't blink. "They are the same thing," she said.

"I know," I replied automatically.

But the truth was more complicated. I had *felt* it years earlier in those Arizona rooms—where joy and grief shared the same space, where one breath could tip toward beginning or ending without warning. I had sensed there was a thread connecting those two worlds.

But knowing it in my bones? Seeing it with the kind of clarity she meant?

Not yet.

Not then.

I told her about a mother I'd cared for at twenty-nine weeks gestation—the day her baby died in utero. When I arrived, she was laboring alone. The physicians didn't come. Stillbirths lacked urgency, lacked "life," and so it was usually the residents who appeared, navigating the delivery with quiet awkwardness, unsure what to say, unsure how to stand in the presence of loss.

I told her how heavy the room felt. How the mother held on as long as she could—as if her body resisted releasing death through birth.

How grief filled the air like fog.

Elisabeth listened carefully.

"We don't teach this part," she said. "They are taught to cure. And to avoid death."

I sat with her words longer than I expected. Because I knew—even if I didn't want to admit it—that grief had always been in the room with me. It was there in that very first hospice room with Ed when I was sixteen. It was there in the ER. It was there in every birth that didn't go the way it should have. I used to think grief belonged to the families I cared for, or to the dying themselves, but Elisabeth was showing me something different: that grief had been sitting beside me my whole career. Quiet. Patient. Waiting for me to finally turn toward it.

I told her about the death-and-dying course based on her book I had taken back in nursing school, how I signed up thinking it would be easy.

"My only intent was to never work with dying patients," I said.

She smiled—knowingly, almost mischievously.

"But here you are," she said.

We talked about my dream of creating a healing center someday. I told her I wanted to call it *NewHaven Healing Center*, after a church my mother's family loved.

"What denomination?" she asked.

"Baptist," I said.

She told me about her own healing center and the people she had "kicked out of her house because they were fakes." I said I'd seen a lot of that in Sedona—how the true healers didn't need to be seen. Their work happened quietly, behind closed doors.

"Don't you think we all have the ability to heal?" I asked her.

"If you get rid of your 'junk,'" she said.

I told her I didn't know what I was doing sometimes, but I'd discovered something: when I touched someone, a surprising amount of heat rushed into my hands. They felt it, and so did I.

She raised her eyebrows, neither affirming nor dismissing—just watching.

We talked about being "helpers" to friends, and she shook her head.

"That's not positive energy. Usually it means being a rescuer." She said it so plainly, but it pierced me. She wasn't condemning me—she was naming something I needed to see.

I *was* a rescuer. I had always been.

"I like to kick rescuers in the pants," she added.

I laughed, unsure if she meant metaphorically or literally.

"First get rid of your stuff," she said. "Then get the proper training. Look at what you react negatively to."

She pointed toward the Rolodex.

"Call Sharon Tobin. She holds workshops. But be careful who you pick to work with."

"How will I know if someone isn't the right person?" I asked.

Her eyes sharpened. "I don't know. I don't know you well enough yet to answer that." That was just Elisabeth, honest.

She told me it took her years to start her own center.

When I told her I wanted to care for people who couldn't afford it, she asked, "How do you plan to finance it?"

I said, "I don't know. I guess I'm praying for a miracle."

She smiled, a rare softness in her eyes behind the curtain of smoke.

On one visit, I asked how I could repay her for everything she was teaching me.

"You can feed my birds," she said, "and get some bread, salami, and cheese—very thin—from the fridge. Put it on my nightstand."

I fed her birds outside first. The desert heat was blistering, but the birds were beautiful—vivid and alive, a contrast to the stillness of her room.

Inside, I washed my hands and prepared her food in little baggies, just as she asked. When I carried it to her nightstand, I froze.

The tray was full.

Not just full—overflowing. Cups, saucers, papers, tissues, small objects, all arranged in a pattern only she understood.

"Can I take some of these off?" I asked gently. "To make room?"

"No," she said firmly. "Leave it."

I paused, unsure for a moment. But then I saw it: It wasn't clutter.

It was her world. Her order. Her chosen way of living.

Maybe care doesn't mean fixing someone's environment, I thought. *Maybe it means honoring it.*

Care doesn't necessarily mean fixing someone's environment. Sometimes it means honoring it.

She asked if I had to leave.

"No," I said. "I can stay." And I meant it.

She had me sign her book. Then I asked, "Will you call me if you need anything?"

"Yes," she said. "I'll call."

We talked about dying—how people know.

"They all know," she said softly. "Even two-year-olds."

She warned me again to get training from good people—then mentioned others who were only interested in money, rubbing her fingers together in a gesture that said more than words.

She reached for her cigarettes and asked, "Are they in the kangaroo pouch of my chair?"

I stepped forward to look. "I don't see them," I said.

She found them herself on her crowded stand.

I put my hand lightly on her knee—without thinking. She snapped her gaze to mine. "Don't ever touch someone without asking," she said, her voice sharp.

"I'm so sorry," I whispered.

"People in pain hurt everywhere," she said. "And I'm liable to karate chop you."

After the lesson, she softened and held out her finger.

"I do E.T. touches."

Relieved, I touched my finger to hers.

"Anything else?" I asked.

"Yes. Take me into the bathroom so I can wash my face."

I froze for a second—terrified of hurting her, terrified of touching her without permission, terrified of doing it wrong.

How do I help without hurting?

How do I touch without overstepping?

How do I navigate this small bathroom without touching her or anything else?

But she rose on her own, and I guided the wheelchair carefully while she navigated the turns. After she washed her face and hands, I brought her back to her recliner.

Here's what stays with me the most: she was the patient, but she was also the teacher. She taught me that help isn't always physical. Sometimes it's listening. Sometimes it's restraint. Sometimes it's presence. Sometimes the greatest care is giving someone space to do what they can do themselves.

"Anything else?" I asked again.

"Yes. Move my commode to the end of my bed."

I moved it. Behind her bed was a picture—a child floating, suspended in motion.

I felt something float in me too. Elisabeth told me she called it *Baby in Space,* a photograph her son had taken. She gave me his phone number saying, "You need that picture for your hospice."

The first time I saw the photograph, I didn't understand it. It's just image of a newborn suspended in total darkness, weightless. No crib. No hands holding him. No background that makes sense. Just a tiny body in a vast, dark space.

At first glance it looks strange, maybe even unsettling. But as I sat with it, I realized why it pulled at something deep in me: it looked exactly like what I had witnessed at the end of life.

After decades of sitting with the dying—newborns, elders, and everyone in between—I learned that the moment a soul leaves the body feels very much like the moment a soul enters it.

A kind of lifting.

A release.

A weightlessness.

A movement you can't see with your eyes, but you can feel with your whole being.

That photo captured something I had never been able to describe: **the threshold between worlds.**

It showed birth not as an arrival and death not as a departure, but both as transitions into something we cannot yet see.

Birth and death aren't opposites. They are mirrors. Two movements through the same doorway—one into this world, one out of it.

On the drive home, at a stoplight, I felt myself pulled out of the present. I wasn't in my car—I was back in that labor and delivery room, standing beside the woman at twenty-nine weeks gestation as she labored. Her contractions were steady and relentless, forcing her body to open when she wasn't ready. And somehow, it was as if her body resisted its own rhythm to release death through birth. As if she was holding on as long as she could. Hovering at the threshold.

Her body was grieving before her voice could.

And in that moment—sitting at that red light—I finally understood what Elisabeth meant when she told me birth and death are the same thing.

Not identical, but intertwined.

Not opposite, but threaded through each other.

Both require surrender.

Both require witnesses.

Both usher someone from one state of being into another.

I had spent my career moving between those rooms: one where life began, one where life slipped away. I had thought of them as different worlds. Two ends of a long continuum. But now the lines blurred. The same skills mattered in both places—presence, gentleness, breath, truth, honoring the body's wisdom. The same courage was required, both to come and to go.

Grief doesn't stay behind at the hospital. It follows you home in silence. Slips into your passenger seat. Waits at red lights.

And sometimes, all you can do is sit with it—again—knowing that sitting with it is part of the same work.

The work of beginnings and endings.

The work of becoming someone who can hold both.

As the light turned green and I eased onto the gas, something inside me shifted. Not a breakthrough or an epiphany—just a soft loosening, the faintest sense of give, like the first hairline fracture of a chrysalis. I didn't have language for it then. All I knew was that something in me was beginning to open.

Not fully.
Not yet.
But enough for light to find its way in.

CHAPTER 16

MY UNFINISHED BUSINESS

Elisabeth Kübler-Ross had a way of speaking truth so plainly that it felt like she was cutting straight into the center of you. She told me many times during my visits with her to "get rid of your own junk. You cannot help other people until you deal with your own. Clear the clutter in your soul." She didn't soften it or qualify it. She just named what I had spent years avoiding—my grief, my anger, the parts of myself I had tucked away behind competence and caregiving. On the drive home, her words echoed inside my chest. My junk. My unfinished business. I had spent my entire adult life helping other people navigate their pain, but I had never sat with my own.

A week later, I dialed the number she had given me. A woman named Sharon Tobin answered, her voice steady and warm. She told me the number I'd used was rarely given out, then paused. "I guess I needed to get your call. There are no coincidences, you know." At the time, I didn't understand the weight of that statement, but I wrote down her alternate numbers and listened as she told me to watch for a packet in the mail. It arrived thick and heavy—pages of questions about trauma, family, emotional history, addictions, wounds I had pushed so far down I barely recognized them. Tucked inside was a flyer for a five-day residential workshop for people who had been sexually, physically, or emotionally abused. For a moment, I just stared at it. I was a nurse. A mother. A healer. Not someone who belonged in a group like that. But the truth was simpler: I belonged exactly where Elisabeth had pointed me.

I filled out every page and traveled to Glendale, California, driving into the mountains with a knot in my stomach. The retreat was quiet and cold, nestled in the pines. The sleeping quarters had twelve beds lined up in a row, like a place where you were expected to surrender your armor at the door. I took a walk before anyone arrived, ate dinner alone in town, and returned to find two women settling in. Liz, from San Jose, had a presence that felt wise and familiar. Chris from Tucson looked terrified, stating bluntly, "I don't want to be here." Liz smiled knowingly and said, "Oh boy. You're probably going to work on some stuff you had no idea about." I knew she was right. Every cell in my body felt it.

Then Sharon walked in—everything Elisabeth had described: warm, strong, unflinchingly direct. She looked at me with the kind of gaze that sees straight through performance. She didn't have to say a word; I knew she recognized the armor I wore.

The next morning, introductions began. What people shared shattered the illusion that trauma had rules. Story after story spilled into the room—abuse so dark I could barely breathe listening to it. Some had multiple personalities. Some had endured rituals and violence I had never imagined existed in the world. My chest tightened; my stomach lurched. Then Sharon began handing out "tools": gloves, a length of hose, and a thick phone book. Before I knew what was happening, someone screamed—a sound so primal it vibrated the walls—and slammed the phone book into the ground. Another scream followed. And another. Rage erupted all around me.

My fight-or-flight instinct chose flight. I stood up, ready to bolt. Sharon saw it immediately.

"If you leave, you'll never deal with your own shit, Leann," she said.

Her voice wasn't cruel. It was truth with its sleeves rolled up.

"I can't stay in this," I said, shaking. "If there's a hell, I'm sitting in it."

She pointed to the door and said, "Go outside. But come back in five minutes."

I walked out into the cold air and gulped it in like oxygen. When five minutes passed, I walked back in. My legs carried me against my own will, against the pounding of my heart. And the work began.

My first session was with Shannon. She guided me toward emotions I had kept sealed inside—anger about men, about strength, about my father and the drinking that had colored my childhood. I swung the hose, beat the phone books, screamed until something inside me cracked. Pain I didn't know I still carried rose like smoke from a long-smoldering fire.

During small group later, Carol looked directly at me and said, "I didn't like you at first. You felt like an observer." She wasn't wrong. I had spent my life standing just outside my own feelings, rescuing others while hiding myself. "I'm no different than anyone else in here," I told her. "We all have our stuff." Something softened between us in that moment—a small healing of the distance I kept around me.

My hardest work came with John. I told him the screaming around me made me feel like I was going crazy. I felt like I was crawling out of my skin. He didn't flinch. He handed me a towel and told me to pull on it. I braced my feet on the floor and pulled, every muscle shaking, tears pouring down my face. "Kick," he said. "Cry." And I did. Old memories surfaced—the silence I had learned to live in, the vigilance I carried, the protector I became. All of it rose and broke open. I sobbed until I felt wrung out. Through all of it, he stayed steady. "You are safe," he said. Nobody had ever said those words to me in a way that my body believed.

Later that day, Sharon pulled me aside. "You're arrogant," she said flatly. "Like me. Like Elisabeth. You could be a great teacher, but you have to let your

Let your heart speak, not your head.

heart speak, not your head." I didn't know whether to thank her or collapse. On the last day, she asked me to come forward and share my story. I lay down at her instruction, surrounded by the other participants. They placed gentle hands on me and began to sing "You Are My Sunshine." Their voices cracked something wide open. For the first time in my life, I wasn't the caregiver. I was the one being held.

It was during that session that I met the little girl inside me—my inner child. Annie Mae. She was small and scared, tender and resilient. She was me before the protecting began. And I held her—really held her—for the first time.

After the workshop ended, I went home feeling raw and unsteady, haunted by dreams and overwhelmed by everything that had surfaced. I went to see Darlene, my therapist, certain she would congratulate me for doing the work. Instead, she leaned back and said, "That training sounds like it came out of the seventies." And she wasn't wrong. I explained what we'd done—screaming, externalizing, acting out trauma. Elisabeth's lineage was intense and unfiltered—born of a different era, designed to bypass the intellect and force emotions violently to the surface.

Looking back, I can say this clearly: not all of it was wise. Not all of it was safe. And not all of it is how I would ever guide someone else through healing. But something real happened there. I learned what it feels like when emotions are no longer contained by competence or control. I learned what it costs to keep everything locked inside.

Darlene listened without judgment. Then she said quietly, "Learn from it. Take what you can. You're doing a really good job, Leann." Her words grounded me more than anything else had. Because healing, she reminded me, isn't found in a single weekend of catharsis. It's found in the small, everyday choices to face what hurts, tell the truth, and soften toward yourself.

As I left her office, I knew I hadn't finished the work Elisabeth had asked of me. But I had begun it. I had opened doors I couldn't close again. And even though I felt exposed and tender, something else was true: I was finally starting to live inside my own life instead of standing at its edges.

This felt like it could be a turning point for me—not just in my personal healing, but in the way I understood my work. All those years at the bedside, from the first breath to the last, I had sensed there was a deeper thread weaving beginnings and endings together. What she told me that day didn't give me new information; it gave language to something my heart had been circling for years.

It wasn't about choosing one path—hospital, alternative therapies, or hospice. It was about becoming the kind of nurse who could hold the whole arc of a life with honesty and presence. This moment was the start of that shift, the one that allowed my work—*all* of my work—to take on a fuller meaning.

I had begun clearing my own unfinished places.

And because of that, I was finally becoming someone who could sit with others in theirs.

CHAPTER 17

CLINICAL HAT OFF, DOULA HAT ON

When regulatory changes and legal challenges forced the holistic nursing work in Sedona to close, my position ended as well. With that door closed, I returned to hospice—work that had always felt like home.

Hospice had always been the corner of healthcare where performance fell away. I didn't have to fix anyone. I didn't have to rescue anyone. I didn't have to be the one with the answers. I simply had to show up with a whole heart—or at least with one that was beginning to mend.

> ***In Hospice I didn't have to rescue anyone. I simply had to show up with a whole heart--or at least one that was beginning to mend.***

It wasn't a career shift so much as a remembering. This was the work that asked me to be present, not impressive. It didn't feel clinical. The lighting was soft, the rooms quiet, and families often brought their own quilts and framed photos that softened the edges of the walls. The whole atmosphere moved at a gentler rhythm, a pace that reminded me that this work wasn't about curing. It was about accompanying.

My shift into a different way of being at the bedside didn't arrive all at once. It unfolded in a thousand small moments—when patients reached for honesty instead of medicine, and families reached for comfort instead of answers. Little by little, I began to notice the moments when the "nurse hat" slipped off without me meaning to—when I listened more than I assessed, when I reached for a hand instead of a stethoscope, when I trusted what I sensed instead of what I could measure. Something in me was softening, widening, making room.

And then came a moment that showed me, without question, what this shift looked like in real life.

I met this Air Force veteran a couple of times before, but on this particular day, the staff told me he was declining. His breathing was shallow. He was refusing his nebulizer treatments and turning down morphine that could have eased the work of each breath. He was "too weak to pick up a coffee cup," he said. "And I'm not drinking it with a straw."

"I get it," I told him. "Do you think if we set you up in your bed, I could help you enjoy a cup of coffee?"

He shrugged. "I don't know."

I completed his assessment in that quiet, familiar rhythm of hospice nursing—offering options, turning him gently, checking his skin, making sure he was as comfortable as possible. Every move cost him energy he didn't have. Even keeping his eyelids open was a battle. His only request that afternoon was a glass of water and some Sprite. We sat him up, he sipped a little, and that was all he could manage.

As I left his room, he gave me a small finger wave. I stepped out to the desk to speak with staff, but I felt something—a tug. A doula tug. That gentle inner pull that says, *Go back.*

So I did.

I returned with a soft knock, knelt so I could be at his eye level, and asked, "Jim, you're refusing your nebulizer, refusing morphine, eating very little. Are you feeling like you're dying?"

He looked at me without hesitation, his voice barely above a whisper.

"I hope so," he said. "Tonight would be good."

I smiled softly. "We don't usually get to choose our exact time, but this is your journey. You get to decide what you want and what you don't want—especially while you're still able to make those choices. So let's talk about what's next. Is there anything left undone?"

He shook his head, breath catching.

"Anything left unsaid?"

Another quiet no.

"Can I call anyone? Anyone you'd like to see or talk to?"

Again, he shook his head. "I've done all of that."

"Okay, buddy," I said gently. "If that changes, let us know. Someone will be here tomorrow, and I'll be back Friday."

He thanked me—not for anything heroic, but for giving him permission to be in charge of his own ending.

He didn't die that night.

But he died the next night—his own way, in his own room, in his own bed.

Alone.

Just how he directed.

One of the patients who taught me what presence really meant was a man dying at home whose anxiety surged every time the hospice team left his room. His daughter asked for someone "different"—someone who could sit with him without turning him into a checklist of tasks. When I arrived, the house was dim and quiet, the kind of quiet that hums with dread.

His room was crowded with equipment: an oxygen concentrator thumping rhythmically in the corner, medication bottles lined along the bedside table, the head of the bed raised high to help him breathe. He was small in the blankets, his eyes darting to the door each time someone moved, as if afraid he'd be left alone again.

I knelt beside him so we were level. "Your daughter tells me you feel anxious when everyone leaves," I said gently.

"Yes," he whispered. Even that one syllable shook.

I placed my left hand over his heart—his chest rising too fast under my palm—and wrapped my right hand around his. He clutched me with surprising strength, as if trying to anchor himself to the earth.

I assumed combat trauma or old war memories rising up. But when I asked what he was afraid of, he didn't hesitate.

"I was a bad person," he whispered. "I did a lot of wrong." His voice cracked, and tears spilled sideways onto the pillow. I waited. Silence can open doors words cannot.

He told me about stealing, about drugs, about hurting people he wished he hadn't. Regrets he had never said aloud to anyone—not even his family—came pouring out. Every confession carried fifty years of weight.

I noticed a small cross hanging by the window. "Are you a Christian?" I asked softly.

He nodded, tears still sliding down his temples.

"Would you like me to pray with you?"

"Yes," he said, barely audible.

So I prayed. Not a scripted prayer. Not a polished one. A simple prayer of release. A prayer naming that regret is not the sum of a life. A prayer asking for peace to fill the places fear had taken.

When we finished, he took two deep breaths—slow, steady, different.

Then he looked at his oxygen tubing and whispered, "Can I take this off?"

"If you want to," I said. "You're in charge."

He nodded again and removed the oxygen cannula with shaky hands. It was the final act of letting go, the moment he gave himself permission to stop fighting.

"Is there anything left undone or unsaid?" I asked.

He closed his eyes. "No," he said. "Not anymore."

When his daughter returned, she sat beside him and told him all the things he had never believed about himself: that he had been loving, generous, protective. That he had been a good father. A good man. She called him her best friend, told him they were more alike than he ever knew, and rested her forehead against his as she whispered, "I've always known who you really are."

His breath softened. His shoulders relaxed. The weight he'd carried for decades finally slid off.

He died two days later, peacefully.

In that room, with his hand in mine and his truths spoken into the air, I felt it clearly: I wasn't there as a clinician. I was there as a companion. A steady presence as he crossed a threshold that terrified him.

Moments like that loosened something inside me.
Something that had been held too tightly for too long.

Another day in the heavy Arizona heat, I visited a man named Dean. Before getting out of the car, something nudged me to bring my wallet into the house—something I never did while working. His wife met me at the gate, her voice tight with worry. She had been caring for him for years, long past the point where one person should have to carry that kind of weight alone.

Inside, the house was dim and quiet except for the sound of him breathing—slow, labored, the kind of breathing you know is borrowed time. Dean sat in his recliner wearing an Army hat that looked almost too large for his thinning frame. The brim shadowed his eyes, but when he looked up at me, his gaze was sharp, guarded, as if he were deciding whether or not he could trust me.

"Where did you serve?" I asked gently.

"Vietnam," he said. Then his voice faltered. "I . . . killed a lot of people."

He said it quickly, like ripping off a bandage, but his eyes didn't move. When I didn't flinch or recoil, he went on—describing his skill, the way it had earned him another tour, more killing. He was searching my face for judgment, for rejection, for anything that would confirm the guilt he had carried for decades. His wife stood behind me, holding her breath.

I knelt beside his chair so we were eye-level. "Dean," I said softly, "you did what you were trained to do in a kill-or-be-killed situation. You did exactly what your country asked of you."

A tear rolled down his cheek. Another followed. His wife exhaled behind me, a sound like a lifetime of waiting.

I noticed then that his Army hat was well-worn: the fabric creased from years of being handled, the stitching frayed near the edges. It wasn't just a hat. It was his history, his pain, his pride, and his shame all stitched together. Men like Dean don't talk about the heavy parts. They carry them until the weight becomes part of their posture.

"No one ever welcomed us home. When we came back from Vietnam, we were spit on." A tear rolled down his cheek.

In that moment, I remembered my wallet and the nudge to bring it inside.

I carried a small American flag pin for moments like this—moments when a man needed to hear something he should have been told a long time ago. Dean took off his hat with trembling hands and handed it to me.

I pinned the tiny flag to the brim, smoothing the fabric as if blessing it. Then I placed his hand over the bill of his cap and laid mine gently over his.

"Welcome home," I said.

He closed his eyes. A deep, shuddering breath left his body, as if something heavy had finally been allowed to slip from his shoulders. His wife began to cry softly behind me, one hand pressed to her mouth. She mouthed, "Thank you," but it wasn't for me. It was for the moment. For the witnessing. For the release she had tried to offer him for years but couldn't reach.

Dean didn't speak another word, but he didn't need to. Everything he had ever needed to say was in the way his body softened, in the way his breathing calmed, in the way his hand loosened beneath mine. Sometimes healing arrives quietly, with no medical intervention at all—only the dignity of being seen.

It was in moments like this—not the charting or the vitals or the protocols—when I realized my role had shifted. I wasn't there to treat him.

I was there to honor him.

And that's when the clinical hat slipped just a little further from my head.

The more I sat with men like Dean, and with daughters who whispered forgiveness into their fathers' final hours, the more something in me began to shift. It wasn't dramatic. It was the steady softening that comes when truth is allowed to rise without being managed. I found myself kneeling more. Listening longer. Allowing silence to do what words couldn't.

Somewhere in those days of hospice work, I realized I was practicing a different kind of care—different but steadier, truer, and shaped by everything I had lived through.

It reminded me of the patient who placed the stork necklace into my hand and said, "You're birthing a different kind of nurse."

I hadn't understood it then. But now, standing in these hospice rooms, I understood what she meant—not a title, but a way of being.

Most people think of a doula as someone who helps bring a baby into the world. But at its core, a doula is simply a steady companion through a sacred transition. Their work is not about delivering a baby—it's about presence, attunement, and witnessing.

In hospice, the transition moves the other direction.

A doula doesn't fix or direct.
A doula stays and listens.
A doula honors the body's wisdom and the soul's timing.

Somewhere in the quiet of hospice work, the stork-necklace prophecy began to take shape. I had stopped being a nurse who performed tasks and had become a witness who tended the moment—someone who held space with the same reverence I once brought to delivery rooms.

I wasn't birthing babies anymore.

But I was helping birth peace.

And then Grace confirmed it, without even knowing she had.

One afternoon I visited a ninety-three-year-old woman named Grace. I knocked loudly so she could hear me, and when I entered her modest room—my second visit with her—she smiled as if she had been waiting.

"I have a liking to left-handed people," she said, pointing at the way I wrote. "So I liked you immediately."

"That makes me happy," I told her. "I want you to feel comfortable with me."

She told how she'd been moved here after her last hospitalization. "It's not where I want to be," she said. "But at this age, I don't have a choice."

She drifted into childhood memories—strict parents, loneliness, and the aunt who lived down the lane. "She let me help her cook and wash dishes," she said. "She wanted me around."

Belonging leaves an imprint. Even at ninety-three, she could still feel where she had been welcomed, and where she hadn't.

When I asked about her children, she paused. "My first baby boy died."

My labor and delivery instincts rose. "Did you get to see him?"

"No," she said. "My mother and aunt did."

"Did they hold him?"

"Yes."

"Did you know beforehand?"

"The doctors did. I didn't."

"What was his name?" I asked.

"I didn't name him until twelve years ago," she said.

"What did you name him?"

"David."

"I'm glad you named him. A name makes him real."

She lifted her empty arms to her chest as if holding an invisible infant. "My arms just ached," she said. "For so long. They just ached."

Grief lives in the body. It remembers what the mind tries to forget.

She smiled faintly. "Then I had Ronald. He filled a need I didn't even know was there. He gave my grief—and my arms—a place to rest."

Every visit with her was like that—heavy with memory, full of meaning. As I stood to leave, she surprised me. She sat up, cupped her hands as if holding something delicate.

"What would you do," she asked, "if you were offered the job of a lifetime? Would you move?"

"Out of state?" I asked.

She nodded, hands still lifted.

"It would have to be a big kahuna," I said, "for me to leave."

She didn't tease or challenge me.

She just smiled—quiet, mysterious, almost prophetic.

At the time, I thought it was just a conversation. Only later would I recognize it as a question already leading me toward what was next.

Experiences like these shaped me more than any clinical skill ever had. This kind of nursing wasn't asking for my expertise. It was asking for my presence. It taught me how to kneel instead of hover, how to listen instead of fix, how to honor the beauty at the end of a life the same way I honored its beginning.

Something inside me began to open in its own quiet way—an early flutter of becoming.

And once something begins to open, signs start showing up everywhere.

CHAPTER 18

COINCIDENCES

Some people dismiss unusual moments as coincidence.

Elisabeth never did. "Pay attention," she'd say. "Patterns reveal themselves long before meaning does."

Sharon Tobin echoed it in her own way, teasing me that the universe tended to "tap me on the shoulder" more often than most. I used to laugh, brush it off. But the deeper I went into hospice work, the more I noticed the subtle ways the world seemed to lean toward me at certain moments—as if something in the unseen was paying attention.

These weren't loud revelations. They were small, gentle shifts. Tiny cracks of light in an otherwise ordinary day. The kind of moments you can miss if you're not tuned to them.

But I was learning to tune in.

The cactus was located just outside my front door, tucked beside the walkway. It was a hardy desert plant—thick, green, stubborn, the kind that thrived in heat without apology. Months earlier, I had wedged a tiny cactus into the same pot, squeezed between the larger plant and the rim. It looked awkward from the start, always leaning slightly, as if unsure it belonged.

Every morning, as I let the dog out or carried my coffee to the front bench, I'd glance at it and think, *I really should repot that.*

But I never said the words aloud.

Not once.

Then one morning, I opened the front door and froze.

A smear of dirt clung to the rim of the pot. A little pile of soil scattered across the tile. And the cactus was gone. Not broken. Not tipped over. Not dragged away. Simply . . . missing.

A clean hole remained, almost too precise. Like something had lifted it straight out.

I pulled out my phone, snapped photos, and sent them off in our family group text. "You are NOT going to believe this," I wrote.

My mom replied, "Maybe an animal took it? Or a neighbor?"

"Mom," I typed back, "are you telling me a neighbor read my mind and knew exactly which cactus I've been silently wanting to remove?"

She didn't have an answer.

Neither did I.

But for reasons I couldn't explain—the timing, the stillness, the strange neatness of that empty space—it didn't feel random. It felt . . . noticed. As if something had been listening to a thought I'd never spoken.

A coincidence, maybe.

But not the last.

It had been one of those weeks when everything felt frayed. My dad had fallen again. My washing machine leaked a river across the laundry room floor. Work felt heavy in my bones.

One afternoon, as I opened the front door to take the dog out, I noticed something small beneath one of my flowers—a limp shape I couldn't quite make sense of. When I looked closer, my heart lurched.

A bird.
Headless.

At least, that's what it looked like.

The image unsettled me. For days, every time I stepped out the door, I saw it lying there, still and wrong. I didn't have the emotional bandwidth to deal with it. Not that week.

Finally, I grabbed my walking stick, took a deep breath, and nudged it gently out from beneath the flower.

And there it was—whole.

Not headless at all. A small, beautiful bird with a soft reddish-orange head that had simply been tucked in the wrong shadow.

My fear softened instantly into something else—reverence, maybe. Or recognition.
The bird hadn't come to scare me.
It had come to be seen.

So I gave it a burial. Not dramatic, not ceremonial—just gentle. The way I honor the endings of people I care for.

And the air around me shifted.
Another tiny crack in the chrysalis.

The group home was quiet that morning—not warm, not cold, just the flat, waiting stillness these places sometimes hold.

Rita, the woman I'd come to see, sat at a small kitchen table. A half-eaten muffin. A bowl of cold oatmeal. She looked up when I approached, her eyes bright with recognition that didn't quite reach language.

"Mind if I sit with you?" I asked.

She smiled, the kind of small, soft smile that is its own yes. Her tablemate, another woman, nodded enthusiastically. "Sit! Please." So I did.

We chatted gently—small talk, the weather, her favorite breakfast foods.

Nothing unusual.

Across the room, a man sat on the couch watching us. At first he seemed lost in his own world, muttering, drifting. Then, louder: "Isn't she pretty?"

"Look at her—she's beautiful."

He wasn't leering.

It felt more like a child commenting on a butterfly.

Eventually he stood, walked slowly toward us, and sat at the head of the table. His eyes met mine—sharp, clear, startlingly present.

"You," he said. "Have you started your book yet? I bet you have lots of stories."

My mouth fell open.

He nodded, as if I'd answered, and added, "Or is it all still in your head?"

I whispered, "It's still in my head."

And that was enough for him. He stood, drifted back to the couch, and returned to his quiet world.

I sat at the table in silence, goosebumps rising on my arms.

Maybe it was time to write the book.

The house was stunning—carved wood, stone floors, soft lighting, the kind of place people build when they want the world to believe everything is perfect.

Vince, the man I'd come to see, sat in a recliner, drifting in and out. His wife hovered in the kitchen, greeting me politely before motioning toward him.

"He's right there," she said. "He has good days and bad days."

I knelt beside him.

"Hi, Vince. I'm Leann. I'm here for your hospice visit."

He blinked slowly, then asked, "Where do you live?"

"Just a couple miles down the road."

He nodded as if filing away the information. Then, softly, with absolute clarity: "And you have one son."

I felt the air shift.

"Yes," I whispered. "I do."

> ***Families sometimes fear speaking the truth aloud. But the dying often understand more than we give them credit for.***

He drifted away again, slipping back into that threshold space where people sometimes see more than we can understand.

When I returned a few days later, he was unresponsive in a hospital bed set up near the window. His hair was always combed neatly when he was well, so I ran my fingers through it gently, smoothing it.

"It's Leann," I whispered. "The one who lives nearby. The one with one son."

His wife stood in the doorway, hands folded tightly. She told me he didn't know he was dying.

I nodded. "I think he does," I said softly. Vince died the next day.

Families sometimes fear speaking the truth aloud. But the dying often understand more than we give them credit for.

As I sat with these moments—the cactus, the bird, the man on the couch, Rita's soft smile, Vince's sudden clarity—a pattern began to form. Little nudges. Quiet echoes. Familiar energy that brushed up against my days with increasing frequency.

These weren't coincidences.
They were invitations.
Breadcrumbs.

A soft reminder that something inside me was changing—cracking open in the quiet way transformation always begins.

Not dramatic.
Not sudden.
Not complete.

Just enough.

Enough for the chrysalis to shift.
Enough for light to slip through.
Enough for me to know something was rearranging itself beneath the surface of my life.

The undoing had softened.

The opening had begun.

And the world around me was starting to make room for whatever came next.

CHAPTER 19

THE CALL TO CALIFORNIA

I didn't set out to move to California. If you had asked me years earlier whether I'd ever pack up and leave Arizona, I would have laughed and said what I always said: "It would have to be a big kahuna to make me move."

Something enormous.
Something undeniable.
Something life-altering.

But it turns out, the things that shift a life don't always arrive like big kahunas. Sometimes they come quietly—like the soft widening inside a chrysalis long before anything cracks open.

That's how it began for me.

Nothing dramatic.
Nothing painful.
Just a gentle loosening, as if my inner world was making space for something new.

> ***Sometimes the things that shift a life come quietly--like the widening inside a chrysalis long before anything cracks open.***

I found myself lingering near water more than I realized. Detouring to sit beside small ponds. Choosing routes that passed by any place with even a trickle or shimmer of blue. I didn't think much of it—it just made me happy.

At some point, I even said out loud, half-joking, half-childlike: "Someday I just want to live near the beach and play in the water."

I didn't mean anything by it.
I wasn't making a plan.
But the words felt light, true, and good in my mouth.

They felt like a stretch of wings inside the cocoon—the first flutter.

And in the quiet of that season, a question from an earlier hospice visit started drifting back into my thoughts. Not loudly or urgently—just softly, like a feather brushing past whenever life grew still enough to notice: *Would you ever move out of state?*

I didn't revisit the moment.
I didn't need to.

The question itself had become a thread—appearing only when something inside me felt ready to imagine . . . more.

Around the same time, my work began shifting in small but meaningful ways.

Teaching for the University of Phoenix—something that had started as a part-time role—was becoming deeply satisfying. I taught in the undergraduate business school, working with students in marketing, communications, and public relations. Even there, far from hospital corridors, I found myself drawn to the human side of the work—ethics, presence, the way people show up. I found joy there. Purpose. Connection.

Hospice was evolving too.
Different leadership.
Different expectations.
Different rhythms.

None of it pushed me away—but all of it nudged me gently toward a deeper understanding of who I was becoming as a nurse and a woman. Presence mattered to me more than ever. Listening mattered more. The energy in my career wasn't collapsing—it was unfolding.

Something inside was saying, *Pay attention.*

And then the practical pieces began clicking into place with an ease that felt almost suspicious.

The University of Phoenix opened faculty positions in Southern California—a transfer, not a leap.

Same work. Same institution. Same mission. Only the landscape changed.

Within days, a hospice agency near the coast posted an admissions position, specifically seeking someone comfortable with end-of-life transitions "from a soul perspective." A colleague took one look at the posting and sent it to me with a message that read: "This is so you."

Around that same time, Jared was growing into his own adulthood. College was reshaping his days and rhythms. His growing independence was quietly but unmistakably changing how our lives looked together.

Another loosening. Another inch of space opening inside me.

And in that space, a question surfaced—first spoken by a patient, then quietly taken up by my own heart: *Would you ever move out of state?*

I could feel the answer forming before I spoke it. A quiet yes rising where once there had only been a shrug.

Maybe it didn't take a "big kahuna" after all.

Maybe it just took the right season, the right openings, the right amount of courage—and a very steady pull toward water.

Once I allowed myself to consider it, everything fell into place with a kind of ease I didn't expect.

A coastal apartment opened up. The teaching transfer was approved with one signature. The hospice agency interviewed me and said, "We hire heart first."

I packed my car, loaded the U-Haul, held Jared tight, and drove west.

When I reached the ocean, I walked straight toward it—shoes off, jeans rolled, salt water folding itself around my ankles. I stood there for a long time, letting the waves wash into the hollow spaces that had felt too tight for too long.

It didn't feel like leaving a life. It felt like stepping into one. Maybe not fully or perfectly, and not all at once. But just enough to feel light and new.

Enough to feel the wings inside me unfurling into their first true stretch.

California gave me a different pace, a different steadiness, a different way of being in my own skin. The coastline stretched open something in me I didn't know I had guarded for years.

There was room to rest. Room to grow. Room to meet new people and try new things.

And room to notice the quiet outline of a doorway forming—one I hadn't seen before, but one I felt ready for.

The first step through that doorway brought me to a man named Dave.

PART III

THE CRACKED CHRYSALIS

The breaking is never cruel. It's how strength is born. You can't help the butterfly by opening the shell too soon—the struggle is what gives her wings the power to rise.

INTERLUDE

THE CRACKING

Before anything breaks open, it loosens in quiet ways.

A restlessness.
A tightening in the chest.
A truth pressing against its own walls.

Most transformations don't begin with a collapse;
they begin with a whisper —
the soft, nearly invisible line that forms
before the shell gives way.

At first, I didn't recognize it.
The numbness.
The ache that didn't match the life I was living.
The sense that something inside me was shifting, even while everything on the outside looked the same.

But that's how a chrysalis cracks:
from the inside out.
The old skin grows too tight.
The familiar becomes suffocating.
And the soul begins to push
against what no longer fits.

I didn't know it yet,
but I was inching toward a breaking
that wasn't meant to destroy me —
only to free what had been waiting to emerge.

The fracture had already begun.
All that was left
was the opening.

CHAPTER 20

THE DOORWAY TO GRACE

California was the first place in a long time where I felt something inside me begin to loosen. The ocean had its own way of telling the truth—steady, relentless, uncomplicated. You can't hide from yourself next to a shoreline. It has a way of reflecting back what you've ignored.

For years, I had been tending to everyone else's pain—patients, families, strangers on thresholds—but when the noise of life fell away, the question I'd been keeping at arm's length finally drifted in with the tide: *What do you want your life to look like now, Leann?*

It wasn't about needing someone to take care of me. I'd been taking care of myself—and everyone else—for decades. I'd raised Jared on my own, built a career, survived more than my fair share of heartbreak and healing. I wasn't lonely. I wasn't fragile.

But I was ready for something different.
Not dependence—companionship.
Not rescue—connection.
Not someone to carry me—someone to share life with.

My therapist was the first person brave enough to say it out loud. One day, after listening to me talk about my rhythms—work, beach walks, quiet weekends—she smiled and said, "You're ready. You deserve someone who can meet you where you are. Just try looking."

At first, I laughed. Independence was second skin. Predictability felt safe. And safe, up to that point, had been my definition of peace.

But her words lingered. They tugged at something deeper, something I'd buried under years of responsibility: the truth that wanting companionship didn't make me weak. It made me human.

Wanting companionship didn't make me weak. It made me human.

Eventually, curiosity nudged me forward. Maybe it was the ocean. Maybe it was turning forty and realizing time was moving whether I participated fully or not. Or maybe it was simply that after nearly twenty years of being single while I raised Jared—him always my first priority—I was finally noticing there was room for more.

So, one evening at my kitchen table, I opened my computer and created a dating profile. Before I did, I made a list—a simple one. Qualities I hoped for: kindness, steadiness, humor, honesty, someone who felt safe and good and real, with faith being a top priority. Writing it down felt both brave and tender, like naming a hope I wasn't sure I deserved.

For a while, nothing happened. A few messages. A few profiles. Nothing that made my soul lean in.

Then one night, a short, unassuming message appeared in my inbox. Nothing dramatic—just a few lines that made me smile. His name was Dave.

We started talking. Conversation flowed without effort. There was a warmth to him, a quiet humor that settled into the spaces between my words. When we met in person, he greeted me with a smile that felt oddly familiar, like recognizing someone you've never actually met. He wasn't trying too hard. He wasn't performing. He was simply present.

He told me a story about losing a tooth as a boy. He said he'd spent months afterward trying not to smile too wide, hiding the gap because he thought it made him look awkward. "I'd smile like this," he said, curling his lip over his teeth and laughing at himself.

We laughed easily, the kind of laughter that doesn't need effort. And when he laughed, I saw it—the small space where the tooth had been. Something in me stirred, unannounced and unexplainable. *Oh,* I thought. *I've met him before.*

I didn't say anything. I just held the moment quietly, turning it over in my heart as our story slowly unfolded.

Something about that story completely disarmed me.

We talked about our kids, our work, the strange and winding paths that had led us both to that table. I remember laughing—really laughing—and realizing how long it had been since joy didn't require effort. There was something gentle about him, something steady, something that made me feel like maybe companionship could be simple.

Our lives had been shaped very differently. I came from a long line of rootedness—Iowa soil, parents who stayed, family first, a farm held for generations, school unfolding in expected steps. He came from rupture and uncertainty—divorce, loss that came too early, a childhood marked by survival rather than structure.

I had a son steady and focused, finding his way through college. He was carrying worry for a son who was struggling, pulled again and again into systems no parent wants to know.

None of it scared me away. If anything, it asked something gentler of me. I let myself soften.

Not because I needed him—but because I liked who I became when I allowed space for someone else.

Our first date was in Laguna Beach. My car. My dime.

There were other red flags, small ones I didn't name at the time—not because I was naïve, but because hope has a way of dimming the edges of things you're not ready to see. I told myself what many of us tell ourselves when we want something to be true: people grow, grace makes room, and I deserved to be happy.

With him, I felt less like the nurse who had to be strong and more like a woman who could simply enjoy another person's company. He didn't arrive as a lesson. He arrived as comfort.

I wouldn't understand the lesson until much later.

But in the beginning, standing in the California sun with the ocean breathing behind us and his hand warm in mine, I felt something stir inside me—a faint flutter I hadn't felt in years. Not wings yet. Just the awareness that they might be possible.

And that small, quiet hope became the doorway to everything that followed.

CHAPTER 21

WHEN CRACKS APPEAR

Looking back, the warning signs were there all along. I think they always are.

But in the beginning, I wasn't looking for them. I was looking for connection—for someone to share life with, not someone to take care of me. But nurses are wired a certain way. We slip into caretaking the way other people slip into conversation. It feels natural, almost inevitable.

Two weeks in, he borrowed money to repair his car. I handed it over without hesitation and never saw it again. He'd pat his billfold and say, "I've got your money right here," as if the gesture itself counted. It never did. I paid for dinners, drove my car, and we spent time at my place instead of his. These weren't grand betrayals—they were small shifts, subtle imbalances. But small things, repeated often enough, become patterns.

Small things, repeated often enough, become patterns.

The truth of his life revealed itself slowly, like shells surfacing after a storm. His apartment was in a run-down complex in northwest Los Angeles, nowhere near the life I was building. Stories he told about his past—college basketball, a business degree—held up only until the details didn't. One inconsistency here. Another there. Not enough to leave, but enough to pause.

I remember sitting with that dissonance. *Why lie? Why invent?* At nearly forty years old, why present a version of yourself that didn't exist? I wasn't a liar. I couldn't fathom the need to be one.

And yet, I stayed. Because we had fun. Because he made me laugh. Because connection—even inconsistent connection—felt better than solitude. And because, in truth, I was still digging up my own bones—unearthing my own patterns, my own blind spots, my own longing to be seen. The parts of me shaped by childhood silence, early shame, and years of tending to everyone but myself. My patterns ran deeper than his stories did. I just didn't know it yet.

We dated for two years—ups, downs, back-and-forths. Nothing dramatic. Nothing catastrophic. Just the slow, steady hum of a relationship held together more by effort than ease. When we married in 2005, it was a small ceremony. Quiet. Secret, even. I didn't tell my family; I wasn't sure how they would respond to me marrying a Black man. It felt safer to keep it contained, tucked close, where no one could challenge it or question me.

Then life shifted all at once.

An executive from the education company where I worked left suddenly and recruited me to run her nursing programs. "Why not?" I thought. Florida, Atlanta, Chicago—pick a dot on the map. We ended up in Chicago before the year was over. Another move. Another beginning. Another chance to build something stable.

But beginnings come with their own weight.

A new state. A new home. A new job. A new marriage.
It was a lot—more than I admitted at the time.

We settled into suburban life. Nice neighborhood. Good people. Trips back to Iowa where my family welcomed us warmly and I felt, for the first time in years, rooted. From the outside, everything looked normal. Steady. Predictable.

But inside our marriage, small cracks were forming—hairline fractures at first. Easy to ignore. Easier to explain away. I told myself every couple had seasons like this. Every relationship had rough edges. Every marriage carried invisible pieces strangers never saw.

Still, there were moments when something in me went quiet. Moments when the gut—my old truth teller—tightened. Moments I smoothed over because I didn't know what to do with them yet.

Moments when everything seemed "off."

CHAPTER 22

CLEARED AND READY

We were at his boss's house on a Sunday for a birthday party. On the surface, it was ordinary—cake, chatter, small talk. But his boss could not settle. His face and neck were red and blotchy, that particular rashy flush that betrays nerves no matter how hard you try to hide it. I noticed it right away. Nurses do. We're trained to read skin and breath and blood pressure before we ever read words.

As we got ready to leave, his boss made some awkward comment about the future. I don't even remember the exact words now, only the feeling of unease under them. I smiled and said what I always say when life tilts sideways: "Well, everything happens for a reason."

Our eyes met, and he stopped.

"Do you believe that, Leann?" he asked.

"Absolutely," I said without hesitation.

I meant it. At the time, those words felt like faith. Later, they would sound more like a dare.

The next day, my husband came home in tears. He'd been "laid off."

Suddenly, the red blotches on his boss's neck made sense.

"No wonder he was so nervous all afternoon," I said. "But why would he invite us over knowing within twelve hours he was going to lay you off?"

It didn't make sense. None of it did. But job loss happens. People make bad choices. Companies reorganize. I tucked my confusion into the same place I kept all the other things I didn't yet know how to hold.

We told ourselves we'd figure it out. A new job would come. We were in Chicago now—big city, big opportunity. We'd be okay.

The next morning began like any other.

He'd been distant and unsettled after the layoff. I chalked it up to shock. I got up early, moving around the kitchen, starting coffee, mentally lining up my day. He sat in front of the TV while I worked. At nine o'clock, the phone rang.

"City of Chicago," the caller ID read.

I thought that was odd, but I handed the phone to him. "I'll be there by ten," I heard him say.

He hung up and told me it was someone with a job lead. I didn't question it. Of course he'd left his work phone behind when he was laid off, so he took mine and headed out the door.

"Let any of my work calls go to voicemail," I reminded him.

"I love you," he said, standing there with my phone in his hand.

"I love you," I answered, fully believing he was on his way to a job interview.

By two o'clock, when I still hadn't heard from him, a thin thread of worry pulled tight across my chest. I called my phone—his now—but there was no answer. I tried again. And again. Each call dropped into silence.

By evening, worry curdled into panic.

I called Bill, one of the guys from his former work—the same one who had been giving my husband extra money for "side jobs." If anyone knew what was going on, I figured it would be Bill.

"He's not home yet," I said. "Do you know where he is?"

There was a pause.

"Don't you know?" Bill asked carefully.

"Know what? I know he lost his job, but what else?"

Another pause. Longer this time. My stomach dropped.

"I don't want to talk about it on the phone," he finally said. "I told him to get an attorney."

The air left my body.

"Bill, what's going on?" I begged.

"Our phones could be tapped," he said. "We can meet somewhere and talk, but not on the phone."

I felt like I had stepped into a TV show about someone else's life. Tapped phones. Attorneys. Secrets. None of it belonged to the story I thought I was living.

He told me to call the police station.

My hands were trembling when I dialed.

They confirmed he was in jail.

The officer on the line said he'd been "cleared and ready."

Cleared? Ready? For what?

My voice shook. I managed to ask the only question that mattered. "What did he do?"

The officer wouldn't answer. "Your husband had one call to make," he said sternly. "Did he call you?"

I remember shrinking into my body, trying to push the word out through a throat gone dry.

"No."

That sick, hollow feeling washed through me—the kind that makes your knees weak and your stomach churn. The kind you never forget.

I hung up and called Bill back, desperate for anything that resembled solid ground. He confirmed what I already feared—he'd seen our vehicle parked at the police station. My husband had gone in without an attorney, against his advice. Beyond that, Bill refused to give details over the phone.

I had also been on the phone with my mom on and off all day. By then, she was ready to get in the car and head to Illinois. I asked her to wait. Part of it was fear—for her, for what this place and this situation might hold. Part of it was embarrassment. And part of it was simply not knowing yet what I was walking into. I wasn't ready to let anyone else see how unsteady everything felt.

The pieces began to slide around in my mind like loose tiles: the boss's blotchy neck at the birthday party, the sudden layoff, the call from the City of Chicago, the silence, the jail.

It still wouldn't click into a picture I could recognize.

Why would he do this?
Why wouldn't he tell me?
Who was I married to?

Then, in the swirl of panic, I remembered the call from that morning—the one from the "City of Chicago." I went to the home phone and hit redial.

"Homicide unit," a woman's voice answered.

Homicide. *Are you kidding me?*

I think she could feel the despair in my voice, the way I was pleading without even knowing what to ask for. She was kind. She connected me to a detective and passed along my call.

"He's in lockup," the officer said. "He had a phone call to make. Did he call you?"

"I'm working from home today," I said, my voice breaking. "I've been on the phone all day."

He told me that they would have let him try again if the line was busy. I guess I didn't get a call. Then he added words that sounded like another language: "He's been silver-chained and card-wallet ID'd. He's cleared already."

"What the hell does that mean?" I asked.

He didn't answer my question. He only clarified the next step: "He'll go before the judge tomorrow at twelve o'clock. Courtroom 101."

That night, I opened my journal and wrote with shaking hands:

Dear Lord, if I've ever needed You, it's now. My husband is in jail. Good God, what do I do? More importantly, what did he do?

My God. Fingerprints. Court appearance. Bond hearing. Lord, I pray today for strength, for reserve, for guidance, direction, health, healing—for all of us.

By then, my body was betraying me. Stress made me sick to my core. And still, I had almost no answers—only fragments and phrases and a growing sense that the life I thought I had was cracking wide open.

I called my mother that night.

"I just don't know what to do," I said, my voice splitting. "I'm alone. I'm afraid. And now I finally understand what it means when you say 'for better or for worse.' This must be the worst."

Later, I wrote again:

Lord, protect him. Lord, protect me. Lord, protect my family. And Lord, help me to forgive.

Sleep came in scraps. At 3:30 a.m.—the hour that seemed to find me over and over in those years—I woke and reached for my pen.

It seems like 3:30 in the morning is the magic number these days. I'm so sad and confused and hurt and frightened. The what-ifs are killing me.

My sister came the next morning to take me downtown for the bond hearing. I worried he would be embarrassed that she was with me.

He will be so embarrassed, Lord. Protect him. Protect his heart. Penetrate his heart and soul, dear Lord.

We drove mostly in silence. My thoughts tumbled out in fits and starts—questions I couldn't answer.

What if he's angry I brought her?
What if I never really knew him at all?

The criminal courts building in downtown Chicago was gray and looming, a place that seemed built to make you feel small before you even stepped inside. People streamed in and out, coats pulled tight against the cold. I clutched my purse and my journal and tried to remember how to breathe.

Security checks. Metal detectors. Uniforms everywhere. The echo of footsteps in long hallways. I felt like a stranger in a foreign country, with no map and no translator.

Inside the courtroom, we sat and waited. Fifty-three cases came before his.

One after another, lives unraveled in front of the bench.

A man who stole a van with a victim clinging to the roof, who fell to his death. No bail.

A seventeen-year-old boy who couldn't read or write, suicidal, armed, already with two prior convictions. Sent to boot camp.

A thirty-six-year-old with a knife, a rape charge, a past armed robbery. No bail.

More cases. More charges. More shattered stories.

I listened, numb, my body frozen, my spirit hollow. I was a hospice executive—and here I sat in a criminal courtroom, waiting to find out what the man I thought I knew, my husband, had done.

What am I doing here? I kept thinking. *How did my life bring me to this place?*

I couldn't help but notice the judge's name: Judge Bible. For some reason, it lodged in my mind, as if God Himself were tapping me on the shoulder, telling me to pay attention.

Finally: case number fifty-three. My husband.

He was brought in, chains clinking softly. I watched from a separate room, separated by glass, unsure whether he could see me or only the courtroom beyond. He didn't look for me. He didn't scan the courtroom, didn't search for my face.

Maybe he knew I was there. Maybe he couldn't bear to see me. Maybe he was ashamed. All I knew was that I felt invisible—like a ghost watching her own life from the back row.

The judge spoke briskly, reading charges that sounded like a foreign language. Felony. Theft. Bond set. The words circled above my head without landing. It wasn't until I heard the amount—six figures—that the room tilted sideways.

In that instant, I knew: nothing about our life was what I thought it was.

My sister and I left the courtroom and sat in the car for hours, snow falling thick and steady, wrapping the city in a heavy silence. At 4:30, I was allowed to enter another building to pay the bail. No phone . . . that left when Dave did. Just my ID and a check in my hand.

I sat on a cold concrete bench with strangers, listening to them talk about their children, their husbands, their own stories of trouble and heartbreak. I felt stripped of everything—status, certainty, even language. All I had left was shame and a bond slip with my husband's name on it.

Finally, they called his name. I walked to the counter and paid the bond, my hands shaking so badly I could barely sign.

"When will he be released?" I asked.

"Go home," they said. "We'll process him." It was after 10 pm by this time. I had no way to call Tammy, who had waited for me in the car on the streets of downtown Chicago.

We drove home through the snow, the world outside the windshield blurred and white, like someone had erased the lines of my life.

It was after midnight when he finally walked through the door, I hardly recognized him. Thick black marker lines covered his arm—notes and numbers scrawled directly on his skin during intake.

It looked degrading, dehumanizing, as if the process had chewed him up and spit him back out with labels.

I couldn't help myself.

"Why did they say you only had three years of college instead of a degree?" I asked.

He didn't hesitate.

"Because I didn't want to get beat up in jail for having a college education," he said.

At the time, I accepted it. Jail sounded terrifying. Maybe, in that environment, even education could make you a target. It was easier to nod than to dig deeper.

Later, I wouldn't believe that answer.
Later, I would realize he never attended college.

It was the same with the so-called "California record." Someone else with his name, he said. Not him. And I believed that, too. My family believed it. We all swallowed his version of the story and carried on.

I buried myself in the routines of my busy life—work, cleaning, cooking, showing up as a good wife. Court dates came and went. Attorney visits happened behind closed doors. I learned not to ask questions, because according to him, he hadn't really done anything wrong. He'd just gotten the "bad end of the stick."

In hindsight, everything—my home, my finances, my safety, my heart—was hanging by a thread. I was already standing on the edge of losing it all, and I didn't even know what "it" was.

I was already standing on the edge of losing it all, and I didn't even know what "it" was.

That Sunday afternoon, watching my husband's boss's neck turn blotchy at a birthday party, I had said with full conviction, "Everything happens for a reason."

I still believe that.

I just didn't know yet how devastating, and eventually, holy, that belief would turn out to be.

CHAPTER 23

THE LONG UNDOING

Looking back, those years feel like walking through fog—moving, breathing, functioning, yet never fully alive. After that first court appearance, nothing exploded right away. Instead, everything around me slowly loosened, thread by thread, until I could no longer remember what solid ground felt like. From the outside, life looked normal. I went to work, cleaned, cooked, paid bills, smiled at the right times. Inside, though, I was hollowing out. I had been married to someone I didn't really know, but that truth only lived in the corners of my mind, where I didn't dare shine a flashlight.

We carried on as if nothing had happened. Another common theme I've seen played out in my life. Court dates came and went behind closed doors. Attorney meetings happened without explanation. Dave insisted he'd "gotten the bad end of the stick," and I wanted so badly to believe him that I stopped asking questions. Silence became easier than truth. He no longer pretended to go to church or fit into my family. He no longer wore the mask of stability or integrity. Pretending had exhausted him, and when he stopped, the quiet in our house became heavy enough to shape itself around me.

My body eventually revolted. Years of strain built up until one day my heart fluttered, pounded, then lurched into rhythms I couldn't control. I landed in the hospital, overwhelmed, terrified, unable to explain the kind of pain that doesn't show up on monitors. A chaplain entered the room and gently asked why I was crying.

I couldn't tell her. How could I? She didn't know how to sit with someone's unraveling, not really. I wiped my face and whispered, "I'm fine," even though I was anything but. I had been played. I had been beaten emotionally, bruised spiritually, overwhelmed to the point that my body said what my mouth could not: *enough.*

I prayed the way a drowning person reaches for air. *Restore me. Rebuild me. Protect me. Make me whole.* And somehow, in the middle of fear and confusion, my heart kept beating. It never fractured.

During our separation, he asked questions that chilled me—small, unsettling things that landed wrong in my gut.

"Who is the beneficiary of your life insurance policy?" "Do you still keep that file box in the closet?"

Alone, each question sounded ordinary. Together, they formed a pattern I didn't yet have the courage to name.

For months, my life became unsettled in ways I didn't know how to explain. I spent weeks living out of hotels, my suitcases packed, important documents locked in my car. The home I loved no longer felt like home—just four walls I moved through cautiously.

No one at work knew. We were caring for over a hundred hospice patients and their families; there was no room there for my unraveling. My team was like family and would have surrounded me with support, but I kept it quiet. I told only my office manager and the volunteer/bereavement coordinator—just enough, in case they saw him.

My heart palpitations continued. For six months I battled an unexplained illness, test after test offering no answers. My body knew before my mind did—long before I could name the possibility that something, or someone, was making me sick.

I never had proof. Only symptoms. Only instinct. Only a growing sense that my life itself had become a palpitation—irregular, exhausting, and unsafe.

The day of the divorce trial came like something out of a dream I didn't want to be in. My attorney said the process would be healing, and even as she said it, something in me leaned toward that hope. I went to work that morning, as I had done through every crisis of those years. Showing up was my survival skill. When it was time to leave, I met my attorney in the parking lot. Rain pounded the pavement. My umbrella flipped inside out in the wind, and I muttered, "Boy, someone's angry today." It felt true—like the sky itself was echoing the storm I had lived in for so long.

Inside a restaurant near the courthouse, she went over the plan. Cross-examination. Questions. Strategy. I held the white crystal my volunteer coordinator had given me—protection, clarity, grounding. We finished breakfast, walked back through the rain, and entered the building where my marriage would finally end. Security checks. Elevators. The familiar hum of the courthouse I'd come to dread. And then I saw him.

My husband.

Two and a half years since I'd seen his face. He didn't notice me at first. When his eyes finally met mine, there was a flicker—a tiny recognition—but nothing more. No smile. No apology. No ache of seeing someone you once promised forever to.

He looked small. Almost wrinkled. The tall, confident posture I remembered was gone, replaced by something hunched and careful. Whatever pride he once carried had drained away.

Inside the courtroom, the judge entered, brisk and businesslike. We skipped pretrial and went straight into proceedings. I searched the walls for the crest my bereavement coordinator told me to focus on—*In God We Trust*—but I couldn't find it. My heart tripped, panicked, as if it wanted to jump out of my chest and run. I reached into my purse, opened my *He and I* devotional, and let the pages fall where they may. Page 142. I read words about trials being "made to measure," about suffering drawing us closer to God, about tenderness, humility, and being docile in His hands. The words wrapped around my fear like warm cloth. I would be okay.

> ***My life had been held hostage by secrets for so long that even the painful truth felt like freedom.***

The trial unfolded quickly, almost quietly, as though the gavel itself wanted to get it over with. When it ended—just like that, without ceremony—I felt something I hadn't felt in years: happiness. Relief. Lightness. I expected to dissolve into tears, to collapse under the weight of everything I had endured. Instead, I felt myself rising. Walking out of that courtroom felt like stepping out of a dark cellar into clean air. My life had been held hostage by secrets for so long that even the painful truth felt like freedom.

A few days later, I was at my brother Gary's house. We talked about normal things—family, the weather, small stories of ordinary life. And then, as I stood to leave, he looked at me with a softness that stilled me.

"I have my sister back," he said.

The words hit me like sunlight breaking through heavy clouds. I hadn't known I'd been missing. I hadn't realized how much of myself had been swallowed by silence, shame, fear, and grief. But he saw it before I did—the return of something whole, something true, something alive. I felt my throat tighten, a tenderness rising from a place I thought had gone numb forever.

In that moment, I understood something simple and profound:

I wanted my story back.

I wanted my voice back.

I wanted *me* back.

And though I couldn't yet imagine sharing the fullness of what I'd lived through—couldn't imagine writing it, speaking it, or giving it shape—I could feel the smallest flutter inside me, the faintest suggestion of wings.

Not flying yet.

Not even open.

Just the awareness that they might—one day—be possible.

CHAPTER 24

THE STORY THAT ROSE TO THE SURFACE

Healing rarely arrives like a revelation. It comes quietly, slipping in through the cracks of ordinary days. After the trial, after Gary's words—*I have my sister back*—something inside me softened. Not healed, not whole, but softened, the way a tightly clenched fist begins to uncurl. For years I had lived with secrets, shame, betrayal, and silence, all compressed so deeply into my chest that I could barely feel God's presence or even my own. And yet, in that corner of my soul where everything else felt dark, something still whispered: *You're almost there.*

I didn't always recognize it as God. Sometimes I thought it was stubbornness, or maybe a thin thread of hope refusing to snap. But now I know—it was Him. A quiet nudge guiding me toward myself.

Around that same time, someone introduced me to the idea of the last 11%.

A simple truth wrapped in a complicated reality: most people do 89% of their healing, then stop. Not because they don't want wholeness, but because the final stretch is the rawest. The part where the identity built around pain has to dissolve. The part where you release the story you've carried for decades. The part where you face the truth you've buried so deep it has become muscle memory.

That concept hit me hard. I knew I had forgiven—mostly. I had healed—mostly. I had moved on—mostly. But the "mostly" was a shell around something deeper. The last 11% was the part I was terrified to touch—my emptiness, my rage, my shame, the pieces of the story I still blamed myself for.

Elisabeth Kübler-Ross had tried to tell me years before: "You have to heal yourself first."

I thought I could bypass that by helping others heal, by tending to their grief instead of my own. But the 11% theory revealed what EKR had always known: you can't accompany someone into their depths if you refuse to visit your own.

And then came Mr. Oliver.

His room was warm that morning, full of the quiet presence that settles over families when time has slowed. He couldn't speak anymore—his body too tired, his breath too thin—but his eyes were bright, alive with meaning. When I washed him, he moved his cheek toward my hand, a small, instinctive gesture of trust. His son sat beside him, tears slipping without shame. His wife stood close and began telling me his story.

Not the sanitized version.
Not the clinical bullet points.
But the whole of him.
Who he had been.
What he had loved.
What he had carried.
Why he mattered.

Her voice lifted the truth of his life into the room like a blessing. And standing there, listening, witnessing, something inside me broke open.

It struck me: here I was, someone who had lived through deceit, secrets, and pain, now learning to witness truth without judgment.

I had been immersed in lies, both mine and others', but in this room, with Mr. Oliver and his family, there was only honesty, presence, and care.

The contrast was undeniable. Their truth illuminated my silence. Their transparency exposed how long I had carried my own story in hiding.

I realized then that honoring someone's story—giving them space to be fully seen—was itself a sacred act. And maybe, in learning to bear witness to others, I could begin to bear witness to myself.

Something inside me whispered, almost shyly: *I want to tell my story. I need to.*

Hospice work had always required me to put on armor—to hold others steady while hiding my own trembling places. For ten, sometimes twelve hours a day, I carried grief that wasn't mine, then slipped into my car and let the ocean inside me pour out. Tears for them. Tears for me. Tears for all the years I hadn't known how to breathe.

But something shifted after Mr. Oliver. My emptiness—the part I used to hate—became the very thing that allowed me to see others, to feel the unspoken weight in their bodies before they ever said a word. I recognized the waiting in them because I had waited for myself for over a decade. A decade-long pregnancy of soul.

This, I realized, was the 11%.
Not the whole journey.
Not the healing itself.
But the moment of surfacing—the willingness to let the untold rise.

> ***Deep shame. Old secrets. Regrets carried like stones. And when someone felt safe enough to speak them—to hand over their truth without fear—the relief was profound. I saw it in their eyes, in their breath, in their release.***

I began noticing how often people approached death with burdens unfinished, the same way many of us approach life. Deep shame. Old secrets. Regrets carried like stones. And when someone felt safe enough to speak them—to hand over their truth without fear—the relief was profound. I saw it in their eyes, in their breath, in their release.

And I saw myself in them.

Elisabeth Kübler-Ross's voice returned:

"Heal yourself first."
Not fully. Not perfectly.
But honestly.
Tenderly.
Willingly.

In those months, the 11% work became the quiet path back to myself. Not dramatic, not cinematic—just small, faithful choices. Drinking water. Walking. Mindful choices, positivity, quietness. Avoiding television. Naming things I had silenced. Letting God whisper into the places I'd barricaded. Allowing myself to breathe again.

Growth wasn't loud.
It was the quiet untangling from what no longer fit.
The shedding of old identities.
The slow return to authenticity.
The gentle cracking of a shell I had worn for so long I believed it was skin.

One day, after a hospice shift, I sat alone in my car and felt something stir—an impulse, a pull, a longing that rose from deep within:

Tell your story.
Not for revenge.
Not for validation.

But because truth wants light.

And because someone else might need the permission you never had.

I wasn't ready yet. But I knew the day would come.

This chapter of my life ended in quiet readiness. A softening. A beginning. The cocoon cracking, letting in the first hint of air.

I walked out of that season with one truth resting gently in my hands: healing doesn't destroy—it births.

The breaking open is not the end; it is the first breath of becoming.

The breaking open is not the end; it is the first breath of becoming.

I was ready to emerge.

PART IV

THE SACRED SHIFT

When the time comes, she doesn't rush.
She unfolds—slowly, deliberately—
carrying the memory of what it took
to become. Flight is just another way of
remembering where she began.

INTERLUDE

INTO DEEP WATERS

A whale spends most of its life in the deep—quiet, vast, heavy with pressure. Yet it must surface to breathe, to survive.

Grief is like that deep water. You descend into it after loss, sometimes slowly, sometimes all at once. It's dark down there, disorienting. Hard to know how far you've gone or how long you'll stay.

And then—something rises.
You.
A moment of breath.
A laugh you didn't expect.
A memory that doesn't crush you.

You come up, and you breathe. Not because the grief is gone, but because you're still alive inside it.

And like whales, you go back down.
The deep becomes familiar.
But each time you surface, you remember: you are capable of returning to air.

One day, the dives won't be so deep.
One day, you'll stay at the surface longer.
Grief doesn't leave—but you learn its rhythm.

And like the whale,
you learn to move with it.

CHAPTER 25

THE WHOLE-HEARTED, WHOLE-BODY NURSE

There comes a time in a person's life when all the threads—every wound, every lesson, every grief-soaked moment—begin to weave themselves into something whole. For me, that time didn't arrive with fanfare. It came quietly, almost shyly, after years of unraveling. The shift wasn't loud or dramatic. It was subtle, like a door I had forgotten about, slowly opening from the inside.

When that door opened, I began seeing my work differently.

I had always entered hospice rooms with compassion, tenderness, and presence—but somewhere along the way, I began entering with wisdom. Not the kind you memorize or quote, but the kind your bones learn. The kind that the dying press into your hands without speaking a word.

After everything I had been through—my marriage, my illness, the trial, the long years of numbness, the crawl back to myself—my ability to witness others had deepened. I didn't just show up with knowledge. I showed up with truth. My truth. Their truth. The truth of what it means to live and die honestly.

Hospice is where truth rises.

Even when memory fades, even when bodies weaken, even when breath becomes fragile—the soul still speaks.

The patient who once told me, "Yes, you try. But sometimes you need to try a little harder," wasn't criticizing me. She was mirroring me. Now I recognize her words as a compass: that striving is different from presence, that kindness is not something you perform but something you inhabit. She taught me that showing up is not the same as arriving.

And then there was the woman with Alzheimer's—some days drifting, some days startlingly clear—who looked at me once and said, "You look pretty today. I love your blue eyes. You have one son, don't you?"

She wasn't reciting memory.
She was recognizing essence.
Her spirit saw me long after her mind could not.

Those moments changed the way I listened. They taught me that presence lives deeper than memory. That clarity often arrives in flashes. That laughter is sacred medicine. That being mirrored is holy work, even when uncomfortable.

> ***Presence lives deeper than memory. Clarity often arrives in flashes. Laughter is sacred medicine. Being mirrored is holy work, even when uncomfortable.***

Grief had carved me open, and for the first time in my life, I stayed open—even when I wanted to shut down. Healing became the rhythm of descending into sorrow and rising into breath again. Like the whales I once watched off the California shoreline, I learned to dive deep and surface often—to honor both the depths and the return.

Years earlier, in Sedona, Reiki had awakened something in me. I began noticing energy—how it moves, how it stagnates, how it speaks. At first, I kept that part of my work quiet. Medicine didn't welcome it. People misunderstood it. Some were afraid of it. But the body never lied. When my hands heated during a session, when someone's breath settled, when grief loosened and rose through the body like a tide—I knew what was happening was real.

Over time, I stopped trying to separate my worlds.

Clinical work.
Spiritual work.
Energetic work.
Emotional work.

They were never separate.
Healing has always been a whole-person experience.

Mind, body, emotions, memory, spirit—they are in constant conversation with one another. Hospice made that truth impossible to ignore. The man who, in his coma, lifted his arms toward the ceiling, reaching for something none of us could see, taught me more than any textbook ever had. I wasn't healing him. I wasn't fixing him. I was witnessing the moment when his soul loosened the last of its burdens. I told him it was okay to rest—that he had done enough. And he let go, not just of life but of the weight he had carried for decades.

Threshold moments like that can't be learned in school. They can only be learned by sitting—emptied of ego and agenda—at the edge of life. By listening to what is not said. By trusting what you feel, even when you cannot explain it. By offering permission when someone's soul is waiting to hear, "You don't have to carry it anymore."

Elisabeth Kübler-Ross told me several times, "You have to heal yourself first." I understand that now in ways I never did back then. Unexamined pain leaks into the room. Fear becomes armor. Suffering distorts presence.

She taught me that being with the dying requires a kind of internal emptiness—not absence, but clarity. Being, not doing. Wholehearted witnessing. Soul-to-soul care.

Somewhere along the way—after trauma rooms, Sedona, EKR, and the long unraveling—I stopped separating the parts of a person, too.

Mind, body, breath, spirit, memory, grief... they are not compartments. They are a conversation. And my work now is not to choose which part to tend, but to listen for how they speak to one another.

I don't think of myself as a traditional nurse or a holistic practitioner. I am both. I am neither. I am simply someone who sees the whole person standing—or trembling, or grieving—in front of me.

When I enter a room now, I'm not scanning for vitals first.
I'm scanning for presence.
For a jaw held too tight.
For the way a person holds breath in their ribs.
For the grief tucked into their shoulders.
For the story their body is trying to tell.

Elisabeth's teachings pulse through everything I do. I slow down. I steady my breath so theirs can steady too. I stand not as a clinician first, but as a witness.

Some days that witnessing looks like adjusting oxygen or repositioning a body. Other days, it looks like placing my warm hands over a tired heart. Reiki isn't magic—it is attention made physical. Medicine and energy work do not compete in my practice—they complete each other. One tends to the body; the other tends to the currents running beneath it. Both matter. Both heal.

I see the whole person now.
I see the whole story.

I see the man whose eyes drift upward toward someone only he can see.

I see the woman whose Alzheimer's steals her name but not her intuition.

I see the patient who mirrors me back to myself, reminding me that presence is not passive.

Loss has changed me. Because of that, I meet people differently now—tenderly, with a deeper understanding of how grief bruises the spirit and how love softens the edges.

And from that place of integration, something I once only dreamed of finally became real.

For years, I imagined a place where people could come exactly as they are—a place where their stories mattered as much as their symptoms, where healing wasn't divided into categories, where no one felt rushed or dismissed or misunderstood. A place where traditional medicine and soul work sat side by side, honoring each other.

For years, that vision lived only inside me.
A quiet dream.
A whispered prayer.
A someday.

Now it exists.

NewHaven. (All one word—because nothing in healing stands alone.)

NewHaven does not live behind a door or under a sign. It is not a room people must find their way to. It is a way of arriving—fully, honestly—wherever the work is needed. I carry it with me into hospital rooms and hospice houses, into living rooms thick with memory and kitchens where grief sits quietly at the table. Elisabeth once reminded me that the location is never the point. Presence is. The work is.

I practice the way I've always wanted to practice. People walk in carrying their stories, and I meet them with mine. Grief has room to breathe and energy has room to move. I blend breath work with education, intuition with evidence, presence with skill.

NewHaven is the embodiment of everything I've lived, witnessed, and healed.

It is where the nurse, the doula, the intuitive, the witness, and the woman who survived deep waters finally come together in one place.

A dream made real—not because I chased it relentlessly, but because I became the person capable of holding it.

When I return to the bedside now, I bring not only my training, but the fullness of who I have become. Sometimes that means morphine. Sometimes that means silence. Sometimes it means breath or tears or a gentle touch over the sternum. Sometimes it means whispering, "It's okay. You've done enough."

I am not just a nurse.
I am not just a doula.
I am not just an energy practitioner.

I am the whole of these things—woven, integrated, inseparable.

I am the whole-body nurse.

As I move through these rooms—hospice rooms, healing rooms, homes filled with breath and memory—I feel something unexpected rising in me: a pull backward. A gentle tug toward where I began. The work I do now doesn't just shape the people I care for; it has begun to soften the places in me that were formed long before I ever became a nurse.

In tending to others, I discover the places in my own story that still want tending. In witnessing their thresholds, I feel the ones I crossed as a daughter, a granddaughter, a girl growing up in a family with its own silences and its own unfinished business.

Healing—true healing—always circles back. It returns you to the rooms you first learned to hide in, to the wounds you inherited without knowing, to the people who shaped you before you had a name for shaping.

And so, even as I practice in the fullness of who I am now, my heart turns gently toward the ones who came before me—toward the lineage I carry, toward the stories that formed me, toward the echoes that still live in my bones.

This is where the work leads me next: home.
Back to the beginning.

Back to the family whose patterns I once lived inside and whose love, loss, and longing I now finally understand.

CHAPTER 26

THE ECHOES WE INHERIT

Home is not just a place. It is a sound, a wound, a memory, a thread running quietly beneath the skin. When I turn toward my family now, I don't turn with the old ache or the old questions. I turn with the eyes of someone who has spent a lifetime witnessing the ways love falters and endures, breaks and repairs, stays present or disappears entirely. The work has changed me. It has softened the places in me that once braced for impact and widened my heart enough to see the people I come from not as characters in my childhood, but as full human beings carrying their own losses, their own silences, their own unfinished stories.

As I look back across the decades, I see it clearly now: we do not just inherit eye color or temper or the shape of a jaw. We inherit the echoes—of what was spoken and what was withheld, of the love that was given and the love that never arrived, of the burdens no one knew how to name. Some families pass down recipes or heirlooms. Mine passed down longing—for connection, for safety, for someone who stayed.

So when my mother calls to tell me that Jared's father has died, I feel more than shock. I feel the familiar ripple of a generational pattern resurfacing—a thread stretching back through my father's story, through his mother's absence, through the quiet spaces where boys become men without the guidance they deserved. And just like that, the work I do in hospice—the work of listening, noticing, holding what is unspoken—rises up in me again, ready to meet my own family's story.

There are wounds a family carries long before anyone gives them words. They live in the silences, in the missing places, in the stories never told or never finished. You can feel them in the body before you ever understand them with the mind. Pain moves this way—quietly, generationally. It travels through inheritance, through absence, through what was withheld as much as through what was given. And if no one names it, if no one stops to look at it, it becomes a kind of DNA—passed down not through blood alone, but through behavior, fear, longing, and the ache of what never arrived.

I've spent decades sitting at the bedsides of the dying, listening to the last words of people who finally want to speak about what was left unsaid or undone. Their confessions, regrets, and unfinished business become mirrors. Somewhere along the way, I began to understand that my own family carried its own echoes of unfinished business. The patterns were not new. They were old—older than me, older than my father, older than his mother who died too young. Pain, when hidden, does not dissolve. It travels. It roots itself in the next generation, waiting for someone to notice.

We didn't even know that Jared's father had been sick. I remember dialing Jared and feeling my breath catch before I spoke. "Honey," I said gently, "Grandma just called me. Your dad died." Jared was forty-four years old and hadn't seen his father since he was sixteen—hadn't heard from him, hadn't received a call, a letter, a birthday card. A lifetime of silence. And yet, in his father's obituary, Jared's name appeared—claimed at the end after being erased in life. What does one do with that?

It struck me then—the symmetry, the wound looping back again. My own father was cut off at sixteen too. Kicked out of his home after his mother died, told to take whatever fit in the car and leave.

He was raised by grandparents after that. At sixteen, a boy becomes a man alone. And now my own son, decades later, carried a similar silence: a father who had disappeared, a relationship that had never been tended.

And yet, the story didn't repeat itself entirely. My father—who had known what it was to be abandoned—became a steady presence in Jared's life. In many ways, he was more of a father to my son than the man whose name he carried.

It is a strange grief—the grief of what never was. There is no funeral for absence. No ritual for a father who left in body or spirit. And yet the longing is real. The bruise is real. The inheritance slips quietly into the bones. Jared asked why his father died, so I went to the courthouse in that small Iowa town. At first they told me no—that Jared would have to come himself. But when I explained he didn't need a certified copy, only the reason, the truth, the clerk softened. She looked up his record and handed me the death certificate.

When I returned to Arizona, I gave it to Jared. He looked at it, nodded, and handed it back. "Do you want it?" I asked. "No," he said. "I just wanted to know why." Something in me broke for him—for the boy he once was, for the man he had become without a father to guide him. I felt tears rise, but Jared—steady, self-contained, grounded—looked at me and said, "Mom, don't. I'm fine. Not everybody has a perfect family. I'm okay with it."

In that moment, my son—my beautiful, wise son—taught me again. He was not defined by absence. He was not undone by silence. He had not inherited the wound in the same way my father did. He had somehow intercepted it and refused to let it become his story. Later, I found myself whispering into the quiet—not to the man himself, but to his memory. "Thank you," I said softly. "Thank you for giving me Jared." For all his failures, he had given me the greatest gift of my life.

Still, the question remains: why do some people walk through life leaving so much undone? Why choose silence when your presence could change everything? I've asked this question at hospice bedsides for forty years. I ask families gently, "Is there anything left unsaid or undone?" And the air often shifts. Sometimes the dying say no and a peacefulness settles. But often they say yes—yes, there is someone I never forgave, someone I never called, someone I should have told I loved them.

Jared's father never had the chance to answer that question. And maybe he wouldn't have. But the truth still lives in the space he left behind. Generational wounds are not always loud. Sometimes they are marked by what's missing—the birthday calls never made, the conversations never had, the protection never offered. Absence can echo louder than presence. And yet there is another truth too: we are not doomed to repeat what we inherit. At any moment, a person can stop the cycle simply by choosing to love differently, speak differently, stay.

When I handed Jared that death certificate, I felt the starkness of what his father had left undone. But I also felt something else—clarity, a calling, a fierce desire to live in a way that does not leave such unfinished business behind. To show up where others disappeared. To speak where silence once lived. To hold with tenderness what others abandoned. The ache of the unsaid and the undone doesn't vanish. It softens. It humbles. It teaches. It becomes a bone-deep reminder: live differently, love differently, say the things, do the things—while there is still time.

And this is how the chapter opens for me now—not with damage, but with awareness. Not with bitterness, but with a long exhale. Because in seeing the patterns clearly, I finally understood: the wound may be inherited, but the healing can begin with me.

CHAPTER 27

THE WOMEN BEFORE ME

Every family has women who hold more than their stories ever tell. Women whose lives stretch quietly beneath the surface, carrying burdens they never name out loud. I come from these women. I did not always know that, but now I feel it in my bones. My grandmother Dorothy—Dovey, as her husband called her—is one of them. I never met her. She died young, in her early thirties, long before I arrived. And yet, she lives in me in ways I am only now beginning to understand.

Growing up, she was more myth than memory to me—a face in a black-and-white photograph, a name spoken softly, an unfinished story. But as the years went by, pieces of her began to surface. Not from history books or records, but from the women who loved her and carried her in their hearts long after she was gone. Chief among them was my Aunt Bette, the youngest of Grandma Dorothy's three sisters, and the one closest in age to my father.

When I visited Aunt Bette recently, we sat in her kitchen talking the way families do when time feels generous and unhurried. Her voice moved easily between stories, memories, and truths she had carried for decades. I wrote in my journal as fast as my hand could move; I didn't want to miss anything. She was, in so many ways, my last living link to Dorothy.

Aunt Bette told me how Dorothy kept her illness quiet. Her skin had changed, her coloring looked "off," and a friend's parents had noticed before anyone in the family did.

Dorothy hid her pain, her sickness, her fear—just as I had hidden my own shame as a pregnant teenager. We were decades apart, but our silences matched. Our wounds mirrored each other. Our way of surviving—of holding things tightly inside—was the same.

I don't know if that is heredity or heartbreak. Maybe both.

Then Aunt Bette showed me a photograph: Dorothy sitting on a rock by the water, her feet in the stream, the current flowing around her toes. Something in me stopped. This is exactly what I do every year on my birthday—find water, find a rock, and let the river run over my feet. It is my place of restoration, my reset, my prayer. And here she was, a woman I never met, doing the same thing. That moment, that picture, felt like a hand reaching across generations whispering, *I was like you. You are like me.*

Perhaps the threads that bind us to the women before us are not always spoken. Perhaps they live in the ways we soothe ourselves, the places we seek refuge, the rituals we create when the world feels too heavy.

Aunt Bette and I talked for hours that day—about Dorothy, about their childhood, about the losses and secrets each woman carried. And then she said, "Come here, I want to show you something." She took me into her bedroom and pulled out a basket filled with heirlooms: a sock darner, lace from my great-great-grandmother, and a spoon. Each piece was labeled with white string and careful handwriting.

"This was my mom's sewing basket," she said.

"And this spoon," she added, placing it gently in my hand, "is the Jell-O spoon. It made it to the table every holiday."

As I held the spoon—its metal warmed from her touch—I felt a strange, beautiful connection to the women who had held it before me. Women who cooked and served and carried families on tired shoulders. Women who laughed and struggled and made do. Women who loved without always being loved back. Their fingerprints were gone, but their presence pulsed through the metal. I felt them.

"Aunt Bette," I whispered, tears rising, "I can feel them holding it."

"I know," she said softly, as if she had been waiting for me to understand.

She packed the sewing baskets, the lace, the spoon—all of it—carefully into a bag for me to take home. I would have left my clothes in California before leaving those pieces behind.

Later that afternoon, she said, "Come here, I want to show you something else," and brought me to her bathroom where a powder puff sat on the counter, worn but beautiful, with elephants etched on the lid. "This was Dorothy's," she said. She used it every day. And when we touched it together, it felt like touching a heartbeat.

We settled into her recliner, side by side, looking through old photographs. She perched on the armrest, close enough that our shoulders touched. Her presence felt familiar, like memory rather than moment. We took a selfie—her protesting gently that she "looked awful," me—insisting she was beautiful.

When it was time to leave, she stood on the deck and watched as I walked to my car.

"Drive safe," she called.

"I will, Aunt Bette. I love you."

"I love you too," she said.

Those were her last words to me.

Forty days later, she died.

Just after my visit, she told my father, "I felt like I was having a conversation with Dorothy when Leann was here." When I heard that, I smiled through tears. Because I had felt it too.

Dorothy, Aunt Bette, my great-grandmother, my mother, my mother's mother, grandma Pearl—these women shaped me long before I knew their stories. Their silence shaped me. Their strength shaped me. Their suffering shaped me. And now their resilience shapes me still.

I come from a long line of women who kept secrets because they had to.

Women who survived things no one spoke of.

Women who found refuge in water and ritual.

Women who passed down more than heirlooms—they passed down courage, softness, and the instinct to keep going.

For much of my life, I thought I was alone in my patterns—the hiding, the silence, the difficulty naming my own needs. But then the stories began to unfold. The photographs surfaced. The spoon found its way into my hands. The lineage revealed itself.

It turns out I was never alone. I am part of a lineage of survival and quiet, stubborn tenderness. A lineage of women who kept their hearts beating even when life broke them open.

It turns out I was never alone.

I am part of a lineage of survival and quiet, stubborn tenderness.

A lineage of women who kept their hearts beating even when life broke them open.

And now, with the gift of time and healing and witnessing, I can see clearly: The women before me didn't just give me life.

They gave me the strength to become who I am.

CHAPTER 28

DAUGHTER TO DOULA

Some seasons circle back on themselves, bringing me to places I once stood—only now with different eyes, different breath, and a heart shaped by everything I've lived through. For years I have walked beside strangers at the end of their lives, holding hands, adjusting pillows, whispering permission into the quiet. I know how to sit at a bedside. I know how to listen for what is unsaid. I know how to witness.

But nothing really prepared me for the moment when the work I offered to others was asked of me as a daughter.

Caregiving inside a family is different. There are no clean lines between role and emotion, between tenderness and old wounds. History lives in the room with us, layered beneath every interaction. What I carry now is not just clinical knowledge—it's memory. It's the echo of childhood. It's the ache of what never happened and the grief for what did. And it's also the love that lived alongside all of it, imperfect and persistent.

My parents are aging—slowly at first, then suddenly all at once. Their needs increase in ways that are both expected and jarring. I find myself stepping into a role I know instinctively—the doula, the witness, the steady presence—while my heart trembles. The professional part of me responds with clarity; the daughter part of me breaks and heals in the same breath.

This is the last eleven percent—the part of healing that brings me back to the beginning as the person I've become.

Some days caregiving feels rhythmic, almost familiar: helping with medications, explaining symptoms, sitting in shared silence. Other days feel unsteady, as if the ground itself leans.

And then there are nights when memory and reality blur.

"Dad," I said gently, "I don't see any bugs."

"They're right there," he insisted, eyes scanning corners only he could see.

"I know it looks like a bug to you," I whispered. "But remember what the doctor told you—there are no bugs."

As I spoke, he looked at me with a clarity that cut straight through years of complication.

"All I can say is I'm sorry," he whispered.

After a lifetime of waiting, the sorries arrive when I least expect them. I don't need to keep score or throw the hard things back in his face—or my mother's. We have spoken of the hardest times over the years. They still ache, but the ache is no longer sharp.

My mother is my best friend. She always has been. We have talked honestly about the hard things that shaped our family. I understood long ago that staying in her marriage during those difficult years was never about pretending things were fine. It was about endurance. Grandma Pearl used to say *for better or for worse*, and my mother took those words seriously. She believed in staying—not blindly, but faithfully—and she carried that weight herself, never asking us children to shoulder it with her.

My parents have always been there for me. Now I get to be there for them. Any scars left from childhood no longer define me; they have become markers of hope and healing.

And it is from that place of healing that I come to our evenings at the table.

Growing up, we always waited for my father to come home before we ate. Now, we wait again—not for headlights sweeping across the window, but for the slow shuffle from the bedroom to the kitchen chair.

Fifteen feet.
Forty steps.
Every task takes time.

I watch him with a tenderness I didn't know I was capable of. The impatience of childhood dissolves; what remains is patience shaped by years of witnessing the fragility of breath and bone. His baby steps measure our waiting, and in that waiting something in me loosens—a compassion rising from a place I once guarded too fiercely.

But caregiving is not only slow walks and soft moments. It is also crisis.

"Mom, are you with me?" I asked one night, kneeling beside her chair. Her eyes had gone distant—the faraway look I know too well.

The ambulance arrived not long after, lifting her onto the gurney—her frail body, her thin breath, the weight of everything unspoken. It was her third emergency room visit in a single week. I called Tammy and Gary. *Please meet the ambulance. I've been up for twenty-four hours. So has Mom.* They said yes. The handoff was complete. Thank God.

As the ambulance pulled down the driveway, Dad settled into Mom's recliner. I sat on the floor with my head in his lap and cried, "What are we going to do if she dies, Dad?"

"I don't know," he said softly, patting my back.

We sat together in silence and waited.

In my parents' kitchen—adjusting pillows, steadying a trembling arm, preparing food—I finally see something clearly: my parents have always done the best they could with what they knew. Their wounds shaped them. Their silence shaped me. Age and illness strip away pretense, leaving the simplest truth behind—love, even when imperfect, is still love.

For a long time, I believed the silence in our family meant distance. But time has softened my vision. I see now that silence did not always mean abandonment. Sometimes it meant endurance. Sometimes it meant love without language.

> ***Silence did not always mean distance or abandonment. Sometimes it meant endurance. Sometimes it meant love without language.***

Patterns don't only pass through pain. Sometimes they pass quietly, through tenderness that never learned how to speak itself aloud.

This is what caregiving inside a family feels like—a slow unraveling of old stories and the gentle rewriting of them.

Becoming a doula to my own parents is not a role I step into with ease. It is a role I grow into, breath by breath. I release old versions of them as I release old versions of myself.

The father who once felt far away now reaches for my hand.

The mother who raised us with steady kindness—the gentlest soul I have ever known, next to her own mother—now accepts help without apology. It's no wonder my dad chose her.

Our roles shift.
The story shifts.

Amid the decisions, the care, the fatigue, come the sacred conversations: what they want, what they don't want, how they want to be remembered. We talk about death not to be morbid, but to be prepared—to protect their dignity while they still have the voice to speak it.

Through it all, there is beauty. I get to be here—not on the sidelines, but in the living of it. I walk beside them as the path narrows. I make sure they are seen. Heard. Held.

Being a daughter is one thing.
Being a doula is another.

Being both requires a heart that understands love and loss as two sides of the same breath.

In this season, caregiving no longer feels like reenacting the past. It feels like healing it. Every meal prepared, every slow walk to the table, every moment of presence becomes an offering—not to erase what came before, but to tend what remains.

And in that tending, something extraordinary happens.

Not because my parents suddenly let me in—we have shared closeness for years—but because the weight I once carried alone is finally shared. I am no longer standing watch, bracing for what might come next.

For the first time, I realize I am **cradled on both sides**—held by the love that shaped me and the love I now return.

Not as the girl who carried silent wounds.
Not as the young woman who hid her shame.
Not as the nurse who had to be strong for everyone else.

But as a daughter who has survived her own unraveling and learned how to rest inside love without earning it.

This is the butterfly.
Not a creature of brightness alone, but of presence.
Of compassion.
Of unguarded love.

Being a doula to my parents is not the end of the story. It is the integration of every chapter before it—the place where endurance becomes tenderness, and strength loosens its grip.

The girl I once was could never have imagined this.

The woman I am now was shaped for it.

And if this is the final lesson, it is a generous one: love is not always loud, and what is offered quietly can still cradle a life.

I breathe into that truth. I let it steady me. I carry it forward.

This is not where the story ends.
It is simply where it comes home.

And in that coming home, I feel the quiet flutter of wings I've spent a lifetime growing.

EPILOGUE

ROOM 107—REVISITED

I stood in the hallway outside Room 107 years after the first time I had entered it. I was there on behalf of the hospice I was working for, walking the corridors of a place I knew well now, doing work that had grown quietly out of a long-ago moment I hadn't fully understood at the time.

The door was closed.

The number was the same.

I didn't go in right away.

From the hallway, the room looked small.

That surprised me.

When I was sixteen, it had felt enormous—heavy with breath and silence and fear, large enough to swallow a girl who didn't yet know how to stay. Back then, I had sat at the foot of the bed, watching the hallway as if looking at life moving on might keep me from disappearing into death.

Standing there now, decades later, I could feel both versions of myself at once—the girl who trembled at the threshold and the woman who had learned how to stand steady in places like this. The room hadn't changed. I had.

I didn't step inside that day. I didn't need to. I had already been in that room thousands of times since—at bedsides in hospitals and hospice houses, in family living rooms, in the quiet spaces where breath grows shallow and words fall away.

And still, I visit Room 107 often.

I visit it in memory, in muscle, in spirit. I visit it when I sit with someone who is dying and feel that familiar hush settle in the room. I visit it when silence grows loud and I know not to rush in and fill it. I visit it when fear flickers across a face and I remember how it feels to be young and unsure and told only to sit.

That room taught me something no classroom ever could: that being present at the end of a life is not a task.

It is a kind of truth-telling.
A kind of love.

Over the years, many versions of me passed through that doorway—the young mother who hid her pregnancy, the nursing student shaken by her first mistake, the woman who unraveled in deep emotional waters and wasn't sure she would ever surface again. Each one broke open in her own way. Each one learned to breathe again.

Together, they carried me here.

If I could sit beside that sixteen-year-old girl now—right there at the foot of the bed—I would place a steady hand on her knee and whisper:

It's okay to be afraid.
You don't have to know what to say.
Just be here. Just breathe.
Presence is enough.

One day, this room will make sense.
One day, you will return—not frightened, but whole.

I would tell her that death is not the enemy. That dying unseen, unheard, or unloved is. And that her presence, even now, is a gift she doesn't yet understand.

When I close my eyes, I can still see Room 107 as it was—the light buzzing, the curtain stirring, the sheet rising and falling with a stranger's final breaths. But now, layered over that memory, I see something else too.

I see who I became because of it.
The nurse.
The doula.
The intuitive.
The woman who learned to sit with sorrow and stay whole.

The one who learned that healing is not linear—it circles back, again and again, asking us to return so we can see with new eyes.

Every threshold I have crossed since that first one—birth rooms, hospice rooms, hospital hallways, family wounds, my own unraveling—has taught me the same sacred truth:

We are never meant to turn away.
We are meant to witness.
To stay.
To love.
To let go.
And to begin again.

I walk away from Room 107 knowing I will return again and again—not always to this place, but to the sacred work it taught me how to do. I return whenever silence grows thick and words fall away, whenever fear asks to be met instead of fixed.

What that room showed me all those years ago is what I know to be true now: *silence speaks.* And when we are willing to stay—*presence heals.*

APPENDIX

Pearls of Wisdom for the Ones Sitting at the Bedside

Before you close this book, I'd like to sit with you one last time.

If you're here, you are likely already doing the work. You may be caring for someone you love at home—learning new routines, following care plans, and doing your best to get everything right. Or you may be someone who does this work for a living—showing up day after day, shift after shift, holding space for strangers at the end of their lives. Either way, I want to say this plainly: no one really teaches us how to do this.

There are important instructions, schedules, medications, and protocols that do matter. But there is also everything that lives in between those lines. The long nights. The silence. The moments when you don't know what to say—or whether to say anything at all. The weight you carry after you leave the room.

These reflections are for that space.

I call them *Pearls of Wisdom* because pearls are formed slowly, under pressure, in response to something that irritates and cannot be ignored. That feels honest to me. Caregiving introduces grief, fear, tenderness, exhaustion—things no checklist can fully address. Over time, by staying with what hurts instead of turning away, something forms. Not perfection. Not certainty. Wisdom.

I'm not offering this from a distance. I'm not standing at the foot of the bed with answers. I'm pulling up a chair beside you. These are the things I've learned by staying long enough to be changed.

The pearls that follow move in two directions: how we care for the dying, and how we care for ourselves while we stay. Both matter. Neither can exist without the other.

How We Care for the Dying

Caring for someone at the end of life is less about doing the right things and more about *being the right kind of presence.* As the body begins its natural work of letting go, our role gently shifts—from fixing to accompanying, from managing to witnessing. These pearls speak to how we honor dignity, comfort, and humanity in the final days and hours. They are not meant to be mastered, but practiced—slowly, imperfectly, and with deep respect for the sacredness of this threshold.

Pearls of Wisdom

Every life is precious—every single one

No matter how frail, confused, sick, or changed a person becomes, they deserve respect, honor, and dignity. Caregiving is not about fixing or correcting someone—it is about accompanying them.

This work is harder than anyone prepares you for

Caring for the dying is emotionally, physically, and spiritually exhausting. If no one told you that, you were set up to feel like you're failing. You're not. This is genuinely hard work.

You will make mistakes

Everyone does—even the most devoted caregivers. Doing your best does not mean doing it perfectly. Sometimes your best will still feel like it wasn't enough. That does not mean you caused harm. It means you are human. Ask questions when you are unsure. Keep asking until you understand.

Giving choices preserves dignity

Whenever possible, offer choices—small ones count. What to wear. When to rest. What feels comforting. Choice restores a sense of control in a body and life that are increasingly out of control.

The body knows how to die

Dying is not an emergency. It is a natural process if we allow it to be. This means not forcing food, fluids, or medications when the body is shutting down. It means understanding that withdrawal and decreased appetite are part of the process. Allowing a natural death is not giving up—it is an act of deep respect.

Comfort and quality of life come first

The goal is not to squeeze out more days at any cost. The goal is comfort. To keep pain and distress low. To preserve dignity. To prioritize peace over prolongation. Comfort *is* care.

Encourage independence—but never shame

If they can brush their teeth, walk a short distance, or make a small decision—encourage it. Independence supports dignity and purpose. And when they can't, step in fully. Needing help is not failure—for them or for you.

Sit with them—without trying to fix

Often, the most important thing you can do is simply be there. Hold a hand. Sit quietly. Let your presence speak. You do not need to fix dying. Staying is enough.

Speak as if they can hear and feel

Even when someone seems unresponsive, many can still sense tone, touch, and love. Speak gently. Move slowly. Let your presence remain calm and reassuring.

Let silence do its work

Resist the urge to fill every quiet moment. Silence is not empty—it is full of attention, respect, and love. Do not corrupt it with words unless they are truly needed.

A Pearl for Professional Caregivers

You may be the last steady presence someone ever knows

If caring for the dying is your profession, your presence carries a weight you may never fully see. You may be the calm voice in the room when fear is loud. The steady hands when everything feels uncertain. The one families look to when words fail.

No one teaches you how sacred that is.

You don't have to fix dying.

You are already doing holy work by staying.

How We Care for Ourselves While We Stay

Caring for someone at the end of life asks something of us—but it also takes something from us. If we are not attentive, we can slowly disappear beneath the weight of responsibility, love, and grief. Caring for yourself during this season is not indulgent or optional. It is part of the work. These pearls speak to how we remain whole while staying present—how we tend to our own bodies, hearts, and spirits so we do not harden or vanish in the process.

Pearls of Wisdom

You deserve honor too

Caregiving is often invisible. There are no applause lines or clear milestones. And yet this work matters deeply. What you are doing is worthy of honor—even when no one else sees it.

Protect them from your exhaustion

As much as possible, do not let them feel like a burden. This means tending to your fatigue before it spills over. Rest when they rest. Step away when you can. Accept help.

Let others help—even briefly

If someone offers to sit with them so you can shower, nap, or step outside—say yes. Even short breaks matter more than you think.

Nobody really knows what you're going through

Caregiving is deeply personal and unpredictable. Your grief, worry, and exhaustion are yours alone. Seek out people who listen without judgment and allow you to be human.

Self-care is not indulgent—it is protective

Eat regularly. Drink water. Move gently. Step outside.

Create moments of stillness. Breathe. Sit quietly.

If faith is part of your life, tend to it. Let it hold you.

Self-care is not a reward. It is a necessity.

Make space for quiet reflection

Protect a small pocket of time—morning or evening—to let your thoughts settle. Stillness allows truth to rise.

Find one small moment of joy each day

Joy does not dishonor grief. It sustains you through it.

Find community support

You were not meant to carry this alone. Being witnessed matters.

Care for your own undoing

As you witness another's decline, something in you will soften or unravel. This is not weakness—it is transformation. Layer by layer, healing happens.

A Pearl for Professional Caregivers

This work will change you—whether you name it or not

If caregiving is your profession, you carry cumulative grief that often goes unacknowledged. You learn how to move on to the next room, the next patient, the next shift—but no one teaches you what to do with everything you absorb.

You are allowed to be affected. Caring for yourself does not make you less professional—it makes you sustainable. If you've seen yourself in these pages, let that be permission to care for the one doing the caring.

A Closing Word

If you are still sitting at the bedside, know this: you are not doing this wrong.

There was a time when I stood in a room like this—unsure, unprepared, and silent. I didn't know what to say. I didn't know what mattered. I only knew to stay.

What I've learned since then is simple, and it is enough.

There is no perfect way to love someone through dying. There is only presence—steady, imperfect, human presence. The fact that you are here, that you stayed, that you noticed, already speaks volumes.

You may never know the full impact of what you offered. A calm voice. A steady hand. A chair pulled close to the bed. These moments may feel small, but they are not. They are sacred.

When this season ends—whether quietly or suddenly—be gentle with yourself. Grief does not follow a schedule. Neither does healing. Let yourself rest. Let yourself be witnessed. Let yourself remember what mattered.

And if you ever find yourself standing in another room like that—one that feels as uncertain as Room 107 once did for me—may you trust what you now know: that staying is enough.

I see you.

This is hard.

And what you're doing matters.

ACKNOWLEDGEMENTS

This book exists because I was never meant to do life—or this work—alone.

There are people who step into your story at exactly the right moment, often without realizing how much their presence will matter. Patty, the nurse who handed me a name on a scrap of paper when I was a single, unwed mother, juggling three jobs and barely keeping my head above water—you changed the trajectory of my life. To Kathy, the social worker whose name was on that paper, who strongly encouraged me to pursue nursing, and walked me through the options available to me. You believed in me before I knew how to believe in myself—thank you. You were both angels to me.

To my son, Jared—my stronghold. Baby, we made it. Watching you grow into the man you are today has been one of the greatest honors of my life. You built something meaningful, had the courage to let it go when the time was right, and stepped forward into what came next. You made being a mom so much easier than I deserved, and I thank God every day for the gift of being your mother.

To my family—Gary, my younger brother, who babysat for a dollar fifty an hour; Tammy, who babysat endlessly and never got paid (I owe you, Tam); and my older brother, Jay, who was already out carving his own path—you were part of the scaffolding that held me up during years when I was doing the best I could with what I had. You may not have realized how much your presence mattered, but it mattered deeply.

To my grandmother Pearl Richardson—steady, grounded, strong, and true. You were a constant, quiet force in my life: gentle, fierce, and unwavering. I carry your strength, your steadiness, and your way of being in the world with me every day.

To my family as a whole—my brothers and sister, my mom and dad—we didn't always have a pretty story. We lived through the good, the bad, the ugly, and the beautiful together. It wasn't always neat, and it wasn't always easy, but we made it. Thank you for shaping me into the daughter, sister, and mother I am today.

To my colleagues, mentors, staff, and students throughout my nursing career: thank you for what you taught me—not only about medicine, but about humanity. We shared moments that were heavy, holy, heartbreaking, and beautiful. Each one shaped me, and I carry those lessons into every room I enter and every person I sit beside.

To the patients and families who trusted me at the most vulnerable moments of their lives—there are thousands of you. To the babies who never had the chance to take a breath, whom I was honored to hold with tenderness and love. To those in hospice care who allowed me to walk beside you as you took your final journey. You were my greatest teachers. Thank you for allowing me to bear witness to the sacred in between.

To Robin, thank you for walking this journey with me—steadily, faithfully, and with deep respect for the story itself. You helped me gather decades of memories, journal pages, and lived experience and shape them into a single, breathing story. Your presence in this process has been a gift.

And finally, to every reader who has ever stood at a bedside, in a doorway, or at a crossroads they never planned—this book is for you. May you feel less alone. May you trust the power of presence. May you know that staying matters.

A SPECIAL ACKNOWLEDGMENT FOR MY PARENTS

This book is written with care.

I am caring for my parents now, as they near the end of their lives. They are shaped by a generation that did not speak easily about pain, fear, or the hard things. Love, in their world, was often expressed through endurance, provision, and perseverance—not through words.

The stories I tell here are not meant to expose or explain them. They are simply the truth of how life was experienced from where I stood. What is shared is done so with gratitude, not judgment; with reverence, not resentment.

Silence did not mean absence.
Quiet did not mean indifference.

What was unspoken then is visible now—in the lives we built, the work we did, and the family we held together. I carry forward the gifts they gave me: resilience, a strong work ethic, and the belief that I could do hard things.

I am proud to be their daughter.

I always have been.

ABOUT THE AUTHOR

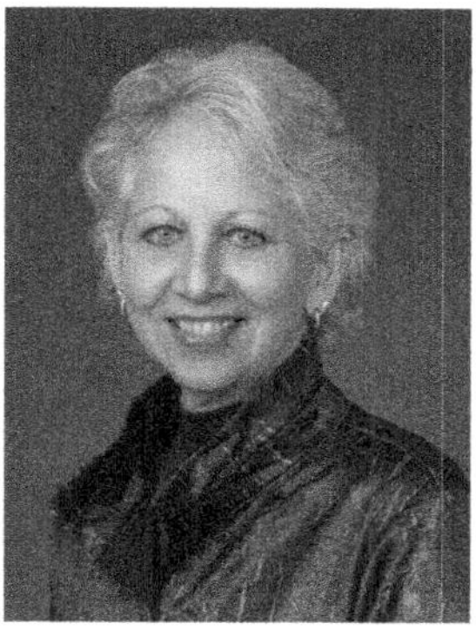

Leann Thrapp, RN, BSN, MA, CHPCA, is a consultant, speaker, and end-of-life doula with more than forty years of experience in nursing. Her clinical career spans high-risk obstetrics, labor and delivery, and hospice care, giving her a rare perspective on both the beginning and the end of life. She is a Certified Hospice and Palliative Care Administrator and holds a Bachelor of Science in Nursing and a Master's degree in Organizational Management.

In addition to her clinical work, Leann is a Reiki Master/Teacher and a sound and biofield healer. She integrates evidence-based nursing care with holistic modalities that support emotional, spiritual, and physical well-being—particularly in moments of transition, grief, and loss. Her work is rooted in presence, dignity, and compassionate witness at the bedside.

Leann is a contributing author to *Complementary and Alternative Medicine: Fast Facts for Medical Professionals* and has written for nursing textbooks focused on grief, loss, and death. She is a Boundless Compassion–certified facilitator and holds a certificate in Moral Injury, with particular interest in supporting healthcare professionals, caregivers, and veterans navigating complex end-of-life experiences. Leann is also a member of the Arizona Nurse Honor Guard.

Through her work with **NewHaven,** Leann offers consultation, education, and end-of-life support for individuals, families, and organizations seeking more humane and holistic approaches to care.

She is available to speak to professional groups, faith communities, healthcare teams, and veteran-focused organizations on end-of-life care, moral injury, presence over performance, and what is often missing from clinical training.

Learn more about Leann's work or inquire about speaking engagements at: NewHavenHealing.org

Made in the USA
Monee, IL
14 September 2026

63221812R00118